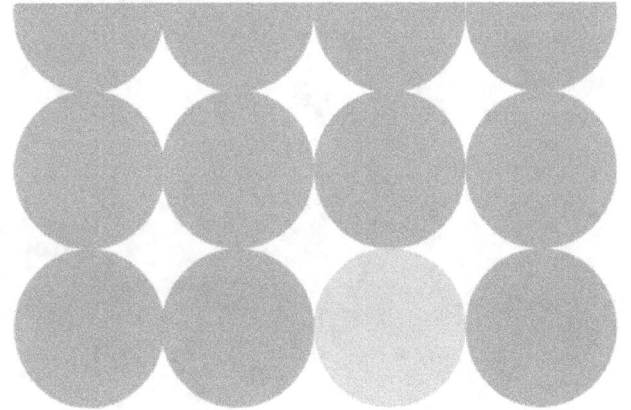

Co-Sponsored by Autism Speaks

I0473751

Workshop on U.S. Data to Evaluate Changes in the Prevalence of Autism Spectrum Disorders (ASDs)

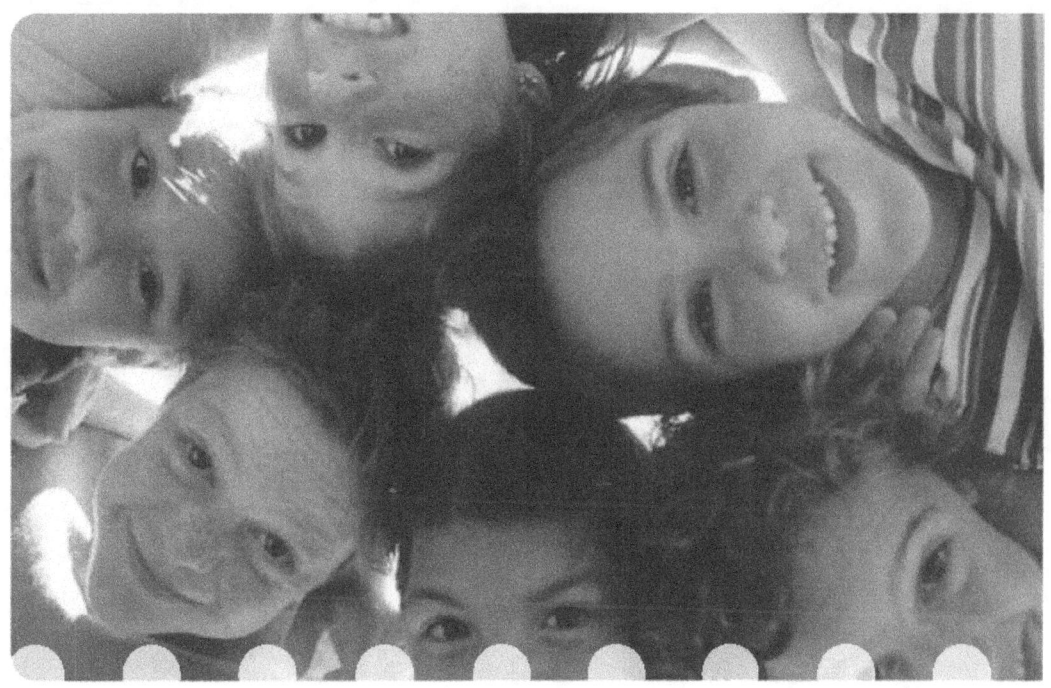

Tuesday, February 1, 2011

Centers for Disease Control and Prevention
Tom Harkin Global Communications Center | 1600 Clifton Road, N.E. | Atlanta, Georgia

Full agenda available in Appendix A

National Center on Birth Defects and Developmental Disabilities
Division of Birth Defects and Developmental Disabilities

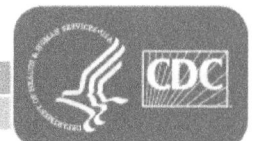

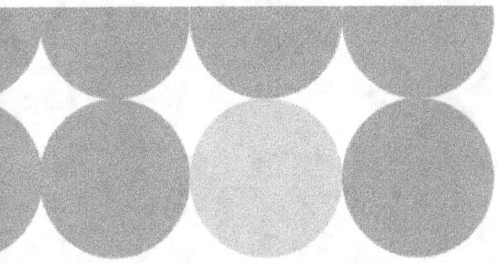

Acknowlegement

Co-Sponsored by the National Center on Birth Defects and Developmental Disabilities (NCBDDD), Centers for Disease Control and Prevention (CDC) and Autism Speaks

Panel members* were representatives from:

Autism Science Foundation
Autism Society of America (invited)
Colorado Department of Health
Columbia University
Drexel University
George Washington University
Health Resources and Services Administration (HRSA)
Johns Hopkins University
Kaiser Permanente®, California
Medical University of South Carolina
National Institutes of Health (NIEHS, NIMH)
Parkinson's Institute
SafeMinds
Parents of children with an Autism Spectrum Disorder
Persons with an Autism Spectrum Disorder
University of Alabama at Birmingham
University of Arizona, Tucson
University of Arkansas
University of California, Davis – MIND Institute
University of North Carolina, Chapel Hill
University of Pennsylvania
University of South Florida
University of Southern California, Marshall
University of Utah
Washington University in Saint Louis
University of Washington
University of Wisconsin, Madison
Yale University

Workshop Planning Committee	
Carrie Arneson, MsC	University of Wisconsin, Madison
Amanda Bakian, PhD (Feb 2011)	University of Utah
Tom Bartenfeld, PhD	NCBDDD, CDC
Julie Daniels, PhD	University of North Carolina, Chapel Hill
Geraldine Dawson, PhD	Autism Speaks
Keydra Phillips, MsC	NCBDDD, CDC
Catherine Rice, PhD	NCBDDD, CDC
Michael Rosanoff, MPH	Autism Speaks
Anita Washington, MPH	Research Triangle Institute
Martha Wingate, DrPH	University of Alabama, Birmingham
Marshalyn Yeargin-Allsopp, MD	NCBDDD, CDC

*Refer to Appendix B for biographies of panel members

The findings and conclusions in this report are those of the authors and do not necessarily represent the official position of the Centers for Disease Control and Prevention (CDC). This summary report reflects statements made by individuals attending the workshop and does not constitute consensus recommendations made to the CDC.

Table of Contents

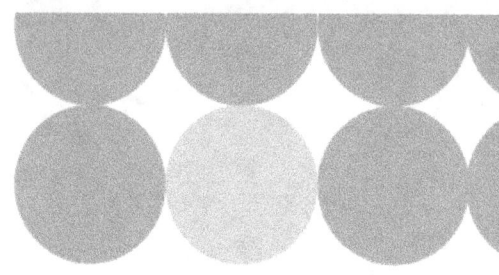

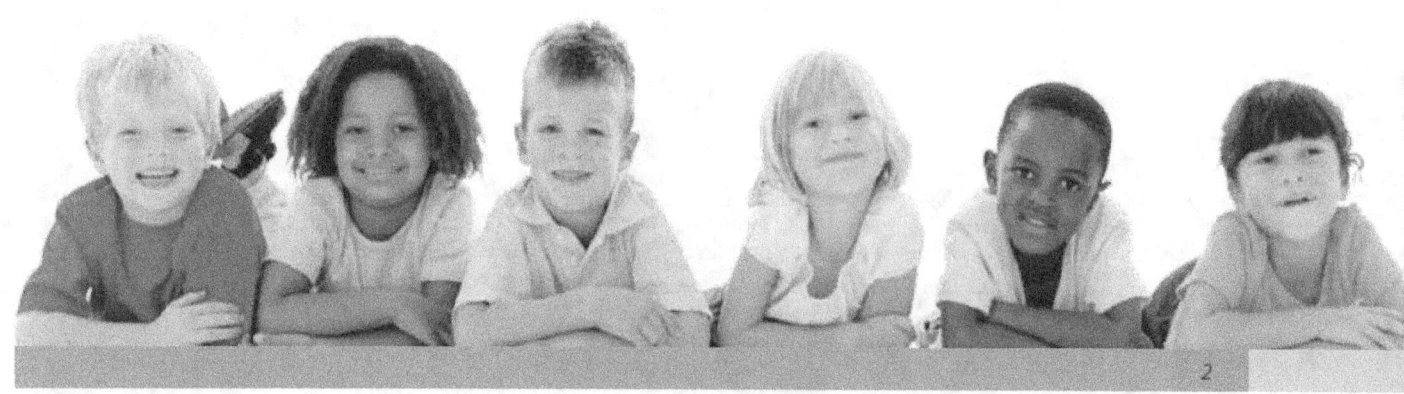

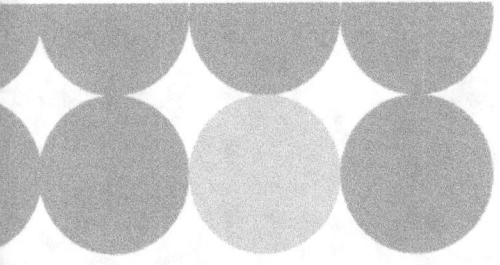

Workshop Summary

PURPOSE

Autism spectrum disorders (ASDs) are estimated to occur among about 1% of children in the U.S. This is in line with estimates from other industrialized countries. However, the identified prevalence of ASDs has increased significantly in a short time period based on data from multiple studies including the Centers for Disease Control and Prevention's (CDC) Autism and Developmental Disabilities Monitoring (ADDM) Network (http://www.cdc.gov/ncbddd/autism/addm.html). Whether increases in ASD prevalence are partly attributable to a true increase in the risk of developing ASD symptoms or solely to changes in community awareness and identification patterns is not known. It is clear that more children are identified with an ASD now than in the past and the impact on individuals, families, and communities is significant. However, disentangling the many potential reasons for ASD prevalence increases has been challenging. Understanding the relative contribution of multiple factors such as variation in study methods, changes in diagnostic and community identification, and potential changes in risk factors is an important priority for the ADDM Network and for CDC. This workshop was co-sponsored by CDC and Autism Speaks as a forum for sharing knowledge and opinions of a diverse range of stakeholders about changes in ASD prevalence. This summary report reflects statements made by individuals at the forum and discussions that were held among the attendees, and does not constitute formal consensus recommendations to CDC. The information, research, and opinions shared during this workshop add to the knowledge base about ASD prevalence in an effort to stimulate further work to understand the multiple reasons behind increasing ASD prevalence in the U.S.

FRAMEWORK

The workshop brought together epidemiologic prevalence and surveillance experts in ASDs and other conditions as well as representatives from autism organizations, parents of children with ASDs, adults with an ASD, and other stakeholders. A total of 342 people registered to attend the workshop (143 in person and 199 via webinar).

Prior to the meeting, the panel members met via teleconference and were asked to submit at least two publications that they viewed as important background reading for understanding ASD prevalence trends. Panel members were provided with the compiled reference list (Appendix C) and articles and were asked to review, at a minimum, the priority readings prior to the workshop.

Presentations during the morning of the workshop summarized current knowledge and issues related to ASD prevalence and provided perspectives from subject matter experts in cancer, Parkinson disease, asthma, schizophrenia, and analytic modeling of prevalence changes.

Following the morning's presentations, the public was invited to provide statements, and there was an open invitation to provide written comments before and after the workshop. Workshop organizers, panelists, and stakeholders were asked to consider these comments when expressing their opinions on priorities for evaluating changes in ASD prevalence.

After hearing open comments from the community, the workshop was divided into four panels:

- Panel 1 – Utility of ASD Prevalence Data
- Panel 2 – U.S.-Based ASD Service Data
- Panel 3 – Autism and Developmental Disabilities Monitoring (ADDM) Network Data
- Panel 4 – What Else Is Needed To Understand ASD Trends?

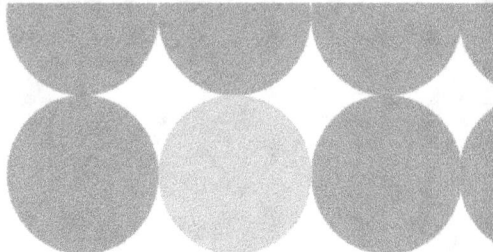

For the workshop panel sessions, members of each panel were asked to reflect on questions along the following themes to better understand ASD prevalence trends:

- What can we do now with existing data?
- What should we do next to build on existing data systems?
- What else is needed in terms of new analyses, data collection, or other efforts?

SUMMARY POINTS

Panel members and attendees commented that the effort to increase transparency and expand the dialogue related to ASD prevalence change was appreciated and necessary to move the community forward around the issue of understanding ASD prevalence changes. Additional key points made during the workshop included:

- The identified prevalence of ASD has increased significantly in a short time period across multiple studies, including data from the CDC's U.S.-based Autism and Developmental Disabilities Monitoring (ADDM) Network.

- CDC is the source for ASD prevalence estimates in the U.S., but other data systems exist or could be developed to better understand trends in ASDs.

- ASDs are conditions estimated to occur among about 1% of children in the U.S. There is an urgent demand to address the many needs associated with ASDs. Prevalence estimates have, for example, fueled action by advocacy groups and the Interagency Autism Coordinating Committee (IACC) and driven the creation of legislation and presidential priority. However, individuals, families, and communities continue to struggle to address unmet needs across the lifespan of people with ASDs. ASD prevalence estimates are important to stakeholders for program planning and making policy changes, in addition to highlighting the need for research into causes and interventions.

- In terms of reasons for increased ASD prevalence, the debate has been dichotomized by researchers, advocacy groups, and the media to indicate that increases must be explained either by identification factors or by increased risk among the population. In reality, a more complex understanding is needed. It is clear that some of the increase has been related to intrinsic and extrinsic identification factors. However, although a true increase in ASD symptoms cannot be ruled out, such an increase has been difficult to prove. Panels discussed needing to identify and use methods to better understand the role of potential identification and risk factors in the changing prevalence of ASD.

- Some people expressed hope that understanding why ASD prevalence has increased may help identify modifiable risk factors. There was debate about the roles of prevalence and surveillance in answering questions about risk and causes of ASDs. Prevalence studies provide descriptive data on the number of people with a condition in a defined population. These types of studies are not sufficient to identify what causes ASDs. However, prevalence studies can be used as tools to examine variation in occurrence of ASDs across place, groups, time, and exposures, which may provide clues about groups who are at increased risk for ASDs. Other study designs would then be necessary to fully investigate the reasons behind observed variation in prevalence.

- There are likely multiple forms of ASDs with multiple causes that are poorly understood. It was noted that sufficient evidence exists that biologic and environmental factors, alone and in interaction, need to be considered as causes. It is not necessary to have confirmation that a portion of the increase in ASD prevalence is due to increased risk in the population to motivate the active pursuit of causes of ASDs. By better understanding what causes ASDs, maybe we can understand the increases in measured prevalence.

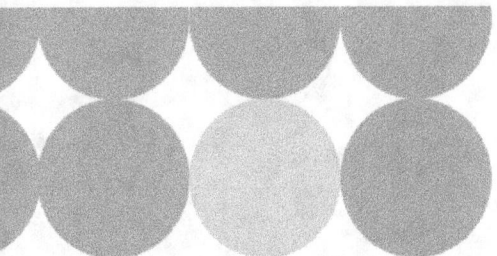

- A risk factor might be strongly associated with ASD and might be modifiable, but it might not have increased sufficiently in the population during the time frame of interest. Therefore, this risk factor might be related to an individual's risk for ASD but not related to the increase in population prevalence of ASD. The model demonstrated that for any factor to have made a noteworthy contribution to population changes in ASD prevalence during a short time period, three conditions must be met: the factor has to be fairly prevalent in the population, it has to have increased substantially, and it has to be strongly associated with diagnosed ASD.

- There was a shared recognition of the importance of, and commitment to, obtaining and using prevalence and epidemiologic information to improve the lives of people with ASDs.

PANEL DISCUSSION SUMMARIES

The four panel chairs compiled main discussion points brought forth by their members for building on existing infrastructure and for developing new initiatives to better understand ASD trends. These discussion points are summarized below.

Collaboration

The panels indicated that collaboration among professionals and stakeholders is important, and the following points were made to assist collaborative efforts among those interested in understanding ASDs and supporting the ASD community through science:

» Continue efforts of this workshop to develop and enhance communication among families, individals affected, researchers, service providers, advocates, and government entities about ASD prevalence, research, and service needs.

» Seek public–private partnerships to support data collection, analyses, and usage.

» Seek input from and collaboration with those in other fields, such as cancer epidemiology, to identify and utilize methodologies for evaluating changes in the prevalence of complex conditions.

» Collaborate with other data systems, such as the Environmental Public Health Tracking Network, to improve access to population-level environmental data.

Analytic Activities

Points were made on better utilizing existing data to understand ASD prevalence trends:

» Provide funding opportunities to encourage analyses and dissemination of findings from existing datasets.

» Link existing datasets identifying children with ASDs to other health, service, and research databases.

» Conduct analyses that will help explain variations in ASD prevalence across subgroups (e.g., race and ethnicity, sex, diagnostic subtype, and geographic groups) and if variation persists over time.

» Use complex modeling and multifactorial analyses to better understand variation in ASD prevalence such as by possible etiologic subgroups (e.g., specific genetic conditions and family history), geogrphy, and sex, and by potentially harmful exposures among cohorts.

» Conduct simulation studies to predict the anticipated course of ASD prevalence.

Data Enhancements to Inform Practice

The panels discussed the importance of using data on the prevalence and characteristics of people with an ASD to better inform service and support efforts:

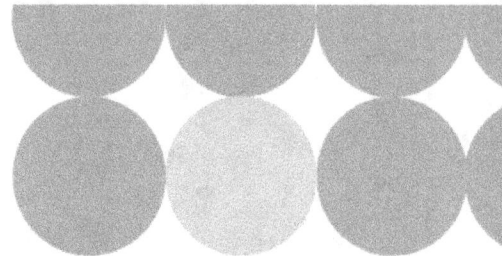

» In addition to prevalence estimates, provide more in-depth information on population characteristics of people with an ASD (such as functional level and impact of functional limitations, subtype, developmental characteristics, and associated conditions) to improve program planning and support needs.

» Examine data to better understand lags and disparities in ASD identification to, in turn, inform screening, identification, and program planning.

» Conduct analyses to provide better estimates of current and future needs of adults with an ASD.

Additional Studies

Beyond enhancements to existing data systems and uses, the panels discussed new types of data collection and studies including:

» Expand ASD prevalence efforts to include very young children and adults.

» Examine prevalence over time among older children by following up with those identified in previous studies

» Conduct additional validation studies at various ADDM Network sites and use the results to enhance estimates of ASD prevalence.

» Conduct further studies to better understand who is identified and who is not identified in national parent report surveys and in service-based data such as special education child counts.

» Develop ways of better capturing the heterogeneity of ASD phenotypes including the complexity of core and associated features that may present in different combinations for people with an ASD.

» Improve tools for culturally sensitive screening and case confirmation among large populations.

» Identify ways to measure and monitor the traits associated with ASDs among the general population to reflect various degrees (dimensional) rather than categorical (having an ASD or not having an ASD) case vs. not case) levels. This includes characterizing how these traits overlap with other conditions and typical development.

» Conduct cross-sectional and longitudinal studies following cohorts over time. This could include examining trends in characteristics of the population, such as ASDs among specific subgroups (based on, for example, race and ethnicity, immigrant status, and socioeconomic status), age of identification, diagnoses, comorbidities, services use, and family characteristics.

» Monitor trends in ASD prevalence prospectively to rule out identification factors by consistently conducting developmental and ASD screening at a given age with diagnostic follow-up and documentation of each step and outcome.

» Conduct prospective studies that examine biology, phenotype, identification patterns, and service needs and use of people with an ASD.

» Examine trends in other behaviorally defined conditions (e.g., attention-deficit/hyperactivity disorder, depression, and anxiety).

NEXT STEPS

The workshop summary will be made freely available to the community through posting on the CDC's and Autism Speaks' websites. It is hoped that the information, research, and opinions shared during this workshop will add to the knowledge base about ASD prevalence and stimulate further work among public and private groups to understand the multiple reasons behind changes in identified ASD prevalence in the U.S.

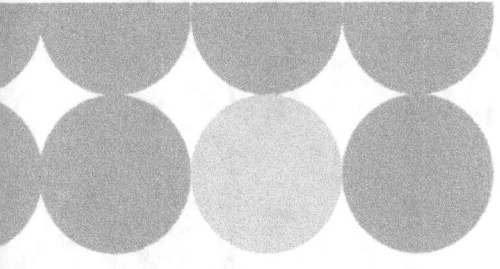

Background and Purpose

WELCOME

C. Boyle and G. Dawson

Dr. Boyle welcomed everyone, thanked the organizing committee and co-sponsor Autism Speaks, and indicated that she looked forward to the discussions and sharing of information and ideas on understanding autism spectrum disorder (ASD) prevalence trends. Dr. Dawson stated that we all have concerns about the increase in ASD prevalence. She expressed her hope that everyone would come away from the workshop with a path forward in understanding ASD prevalence changes and stated that we are much better prepared to address problems than ever before because of better data and analytic tools. These data and tools are from the Centers for Disease Control and Prevention's (CDC) Autism and Developmental Disabilities Monitoring (ADDM) Network, as well as other informative datasets from California and Europe. She remarked that many published papers cite several reasons for the possible increase in ASD prevalence including better analytic tools and broader awareness and diagnosis. However, these papers all have included the statement "a true increase in prevalence cannot be ruled out." She ventured that she looked forward to lively and productive discussion and concrete actions that can improve the understanding of why ASD prevalence has been increasing, with the ultimate goal of addressing the needs of people with autism.

Background: What Do We Know About ASD Prevalence?

M. Yeargin-Allsopp

Autism once was thought to be a rare condition, affecting about 1 in 2,000 individuals. It was thought of as mental illness, specifically schizophrenia of childhood, and was believed to be due to poor parenting. The "refrigerator mother" perception was prominent until the 1970s, continuing even into the 1980s. Today, autism is recognized as having a biologic basis and a range or spectrum of presentations. The autism spectrum disorders have been shown to occur among about 1% of children in several different countries. In addition to the core areas of impairment in social, communication, and behavioral domains, people with ASDs can have associated challenges in other areas such as sleeping, eating, attention, mood regulation, and gastrointestinal issues. It is recognized widely that ASDs have a strong genetic basis, but this is not a simple association and there is increasing recognition of the role of environmental factors. ASDs are now recognized as a complex disorder, most likely due to interactions between genes and the environment.

Beginning in the mid-1990s, concerns arose about increases in the numbers of individuals with autism identified in service systems. For example, starting in the early 1990s, the California Department of Developmental Services and the U.S. Department of Education's Office of Special Education documented increases in the need for autism services. Not all people with an ASD are identified by these service systems, so methods are needed to identify who else might have an ASD among the general population. CDC's ADDM Network conducts surveillance to estimate ASD prevalence in multiple areas of the U.S. and provides data to describe variations and changes over time. The ADDM Network reports ASD prevalence, or the total number of children with an ASD at a specified age in a specified year per 1,000 children in the population. The ADDM Network does not use incidence because incidence is based on new cases where a clear onset time can be documented. Typically, the onset of an ASD is not known, although it usually manifests by the time a child is 3 years of age. However, there is a great deal of variability in when a child actually manifests symptoms and then is diagnosed with an ASD.

There are several potential explanations that can account for an increase in the number of individuals diagnosed with ASDs, including better identification and screening methods, changes in diagnostic criteria, increased awareness among parents and clinicians, and changes in the availability of services. There also have been some studies that have examined how much of an increase is accounted for by other factors, such as increasing parental age. However, a full explanation must consider multiple factors that are not independent of each other. Prevalence estimates are important for planning policy and service needs and identifying promising clues about who is at risk for an ASD.

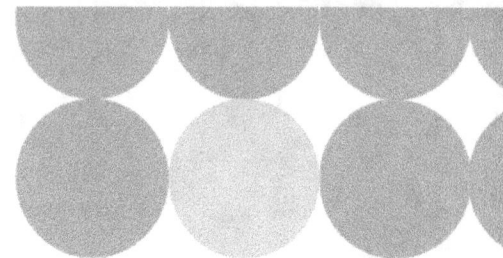

Framework For This Workshop
C. Rice

The identified prevalence of ASDs has increased significantly in a short time period across multiple studies, including the CDC's ADDM Network. ASDs are conditions estimated to occur among about 1% of all children. There is an urgent demand to address the many needs associated with ASDs, and concerns about ASD prevalence numbers have fueled local, state, and national action in terms of advocacy, policies, research, and creation of the Interagency Autism Coordinating Committee (IACC) among other activities. However, individuals and families continue to struggle to address and meet the needs associated with ASDs across their lifespan. Although prevalence estimates can help with service and policy efforts, increases in ASD prevalence beg the questions "Why?" and "Is the increase an actual increase in risk for ASDs?" The implication is that, if there is an increase in actual ASD risk, there might be modifiable risk factors to prevent ASDs from occurring. These questions get to the heart of what causes ASDs. Although multiple, complex genetic and environmental interactions are likely, we still have very limited information on what predisposes a fetus or child to have an ASD, what might increase risk, and which risks lead to the development of an ASD.

A prevalence study is an epidemiologic tool that describes the occurrence of a condition in a defined population in a defined time period. Surveillance is the ongoing monitoring of prevalence in a defined population over time. These studies provide descriptive data on the number of people with a condition in a defined population. These types of studies are not sufficient to identify what causes ASDs. However, prevalence studies can be used as tools to examine variation in occurrence of ASDs across place, groups, time, and exposures, and this may provide clues about groups who are at increased risk for ASDs. Prevalence studies can provide observations that might need further causal examination. For example, prevalence studies have shown that there are about 4 to 5 boys for every girl with an ASD. However, basic studies of the biology of individuals with an ASD are necessary to explain the mechanism that results in boys being at greater risk than girls.

Debates about reasons for ASD prevalence increases often have been dichotomized to point to explanations of better identification or evidence of increased risk implicating specific environmental factors. At this point, although we do know that some of the increase is related to identification factors, a true increase cannot be ruled out—but, it is hard to prove. We also know enough about potential causal mechanisms of ASDs to not pigeonhole the search for ASD causes to only genetic factors; complex biologic and environmental factors must be pursued as well. In order to evaluate ASD prevalence changes, scientists tend to use a systematic approach based on training in scientific methods where the first step is to rule out alternative explanations. This approach begins by examining factors that could explain a difference over time that are attributable to artifacts, rather than "true" increases. This approach tends to examine identification and methodological factors, as these variables are often more observable than the many potential and unknown risk factors that might contribute to ASD prevalence changes. As more data are collected and analyzed and different hypotheses evaluated over time and across studies, additional conclusions can be drawn. Understandably, this methodical approach is frustrating, especially when most people want to know *the* definitive reason for changes in ASD prevalence and whether it is something in the environment we can do something about. The fact that, despite many efforts, we have not found a single, simple explanation indicates that there are likely multiple, overlapping factors contributing to increases in ASD prevalence.

The purpose of the workshop was to bring together experts in epidemiologic prevalence and surveillance of ASDs and other conditions as well as stakeholders to: summarize where we are; learn from efforts to document prevalence changes among other conditions; and improve the specificity in quantifying and qualifying the multiple factors that might be influencing trends in ASD prevalence, including:

1. **Intrinsic Identification**—Internal methodology or measurement factors involved in documenting ASD prevalence trends (e.g., differences in study methods may lead to different individuals being counted or

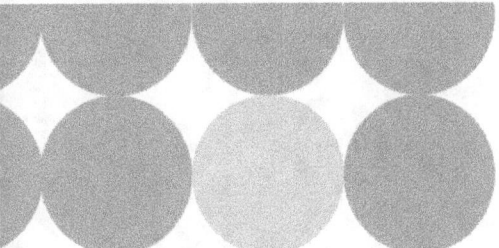

not counted as having an ASD such as using a registry of children identified with an ASD or active screening).

2. **Extrinsic Identification**—External classification and awareness factors involved in identifying people with ASDs in the population (e.g., changes in diagnostic criteria or access to services based on an ASD label may influence who is identified for ASD prevalence studies).

3. **Risk**—Possible etiologic or true change in ASD symptoms among the population in relation to single or combined genetic, biologic, or environmental factors, or a combination thereof (e.g., specific biologic vulnerabilities or exposures in the environment that increase the risk of developing an ASD).

Four panels were formed for this workshop:

- Panel 1 – Utility of ASD Prevalence Data

- Panel 2 – U.S.-Based ASD Service Data

- Panel 3 – Autism and Developmental Disabilities Monitoring (ADDM) Network Data

- Panel 4 – What Else Is Needed To Understand ASD Trends?

After hearing the morning's presentations, members of the four panels were asked to discuss the following questions to provide a better understand of ASD prevalence trends:

1. What can we do now with existing data?

2. What should we do next to build on existing data systems?

3. What else is needed in terms of new analyses, data collection, or other efforts?

The goal of this workshop was to learn from different perspectives to inform the community and stimulate further work to understand the multiple reasons behind increasing ASD prevalence in the U.S.

A Model for Assessing the Contribution of Various Risk Factors to Recent ASD Prevalence Increase in the U.S.

L. Schieve

This presentation reviewed preliminary results of a study to formulate a mathematical model to assess the likely effects that given risk factors had on recent ASD prevalence increase and to apply the model to specific prenatal and perinatal risk factors previously found to be associated with ASDs. According to the ADDM Network report from 2009, there was a 57% increase in the prevalence of autism spectrum disorders (ASDs) from 2002 to 2006. The effect of a given risk factor on prevalence depends on the baseline prevalence of the risk factor (RFP), the change in RFP over time (cRFP), and the magnitude of the relative risk (RR). A number of previous studies consistently have indicated that preterm birth and low birthweight are risk factors for ASDs, and some other studies have implicated multiple birth, cesarean delivery, breech presentation, and assisted reproductive technology (ART) as possible risk factors. However, none have had sufficient values for RFP, cRFP, and RR to have contributed substantively to the recently observed ASD increase. While at an individual level, having one or more perinatal risk factors might convey a moderate or strong risk for having an ASD, these factors are unlikely to explain a large proportion of the population increase in ASD prevalence. Although examples were given using selected prenatal and perinatal risk factors, this model could be extended to assess various other risk factors.

A risk factor might be strongly associated with ASD and might be modifiable, but it might not have increased sufficiently in the population during the time frame of interest. Therefore, this risk factor might be related to an individual's risk for ASD but not related to the increase in population prevalence of ASD. The model demonstrated that for any factor to have made a noteworthy contribution to population changes in ASD prevalence during a short time period, three conditions must be met: the factor has to be fairly prevalent in the population, it has to have increased substantially, and it has to be strongly associated with diagnosed ASD.

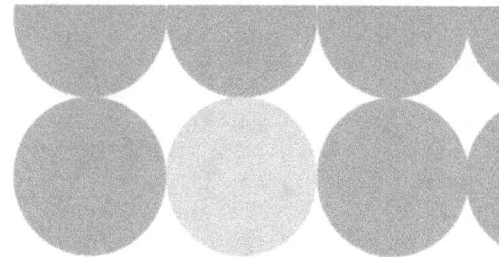

A panel member asked if broad social changes, as opposed to individual risk factors, also were considered. The panel member was concerned that, by not fully examining population-level changes, the model might be underestimating the contribution of the change in that risk factor in the population on ASD prevalence. Dr. Schieve indicated that a large increase still would need to have an individual effect, and the model is accurate for shorter time intervals such as a few years. As the time period gets longer, then a different analytic model might be needed.

ASD Genetic Variation and Gene–Environment Interaction
K. Crider

This presentation summarized how genetic variations and gene-environment interactions could play a role in ASDs and provided background on how these factors may or may not change in a way that would affect ASD prevalence over a short period of time. Typically, to examine heritability of a condition, twin studies are used. More than 30 studies to date consistently have shown higher concordance between monozygotic than dizygotic twins, suggesting there is a strong genetic component associated with ASDs. ASDs have been associated with the following genetic variations: mutation of a gene, deletion of a large or small region of a gene, mutation of another gene, methylation of a gene, or creation of another copy of the gene or the region or chromosome. It is estimated that all genetic variants discovered to date are present in 10% to 15% of people with an ASD and many are implicated in other conditions (e.g., attention deficit hyperactivity disorder and schizophrenia). In general, there would not be an epidemic of a purely genetic condition because genes change over evolutionary time. However, shorter term changes can be seen if there are increases in mutations or breaks, or both, in chromosomes, changes occur in epigenetic patterning (e.g., DNA methylation) or in selective mating patterns.

Gene–environment interactions such as infection, stress, obesity, and trauma all can create the same type of cell damage. Specific causes may or may not have the statistical power to show the true association individually because multiple genetic and environmental factors can lead to the same disorder therefor, studies should be designed to take this into consideration. In some conditions, the magnitude of gene–environment interaction varies. Exposures associated with an increased risk for autism also are associated with other conditions, such as birth defects and cerebral palsy. Single exposures (genetic or environmental) are unlikely (but possible) to show a dramatic increased risk among the general population. Not every individual who carries these forms of genetic variation will have an ASD, which suggests the importance of interactions among multiple genes or gene–environment interaction, or both, in the occurrence of ASDs.

A panel member questioned the accuracy of the statistic that about 10% to 15% of children with an ASD have an identifiable genetic condition. Dr. Crider stated that the statistic is used by others in the field and is a best estimate, but noted the statistic needs better evaluation.

Autism and Developmental Disabilities Monitoring (ADDM) Network
C. Rice

ADDM Network Overview

The ADDM Network is a collaboration of multiple sites in the U.S. to determine and monitor the prevalence of ASDs among 8-year-old children and to track peak prevalence over time. Children are identified through multiple education or health evaluation records if there is an ASD diagnosis, a special education classification, a suspicion of an ASD, or a social behavior associated with an ASD, even when an ASD has not been diagnosed. Clinician reviewers apply the current diagnostic standard criteria of the American Psychiatric Association's *Diagnostic and Statistical Manual, 4th edition, text revision (DSM-IVTR)*. The

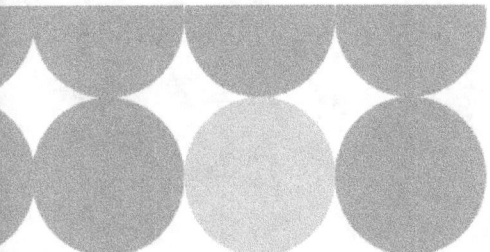

strengths and limitations of the ADDM Network were discussed. The most recent ADDM Network estimates indicated that an average of 1 in 110 children (range from 1 in 80 to 1 in 240) had an ASD and that ASD prevalence had increased 57% over a 4-year period from 2002 to 2006. According to the ADDM Network data, the overall trend in ASD prevalence showed consistent increases, but variation existed among sites and among subgroups. While the increase in observed ASD prevalence at ADDM Network sites could be partly explained by identification factors—such as better information available in records, a more stable population at some sites, and improved identification of specific subgroups such as Hispanic children and children without cognitive impairment—these identification factors did not explain the total increase in prevalence. A neat explanation of all factors that could explain completely the observed increase is unlikely, and further work is needed to evaluate multiple identification and risk factors.

Changes in ASD Diagnostic Criteria

This presentation reported on a preliminary analysis of how an identification factor could be evaluated using the ADDM Network data. Although it often has been stated that the changes in diagnostic criteria that occurred in the *DSM* in 1980 *(DSM III)*, 1987 *(DSM III-R)*, and 1994 *(DSM-IV* and minor changes for *DSM-IV-TR* in 2000) have affected reported ASD prevalence, no known studies have quantified this effect directly. Recoding the ADDM Network data based on the three diagnostic standards *(DSM III, III-R, and IV-TR)*, it was found that autism and ASD prevalence were similar using *DSM III* and *III-R* standards, but increased significantly using *DSM-IV-TR* standards. A portion of the prevalence increase over time might have been attributed to differences in the definitions of ASD used for identification of ASDs by community professionals and service systems. This recoding analysis represents one example of an effort to provide more concrete estimates regarding the effects of a single factor on ASD prevalence.

Panel member discussion:

Panel members raised several questions regarding reasons or theories to explain the wide range of ASD prevalence observed among ADDM Network sites, including the quality of data sources or records and the effect it might have had on prevalence and the inclusion or exclusion criteria used by the ADDM Network sites. Dr. Rice indicated there were some identifiable reasons explaining why the ASD prevalence estimates were lower at some ADDM Network sites (e.g., limited availability of education records) and higher at others (e.g., better quality of documentation in the records). Also, it is easier to identify reasons for lower prevalence estimates than for higher estimates. However, if a site had a low prevalence not due to a methodologic issue, it would be important to consider whether protective factors were at work at that particular site. A question was raised about the reason why the number of sites varied over the surveillance years. Dr. Rice explained that the number of ADDM Network sites depends on available funding and that sites go through a competitive application process in which the applicant must demonstrate a minimum population, partnerships with health departments, and other criteria based on independent peer review. A panel member also questioned when CDC was going to take the issue of rising ASD prevalence seriously. Dr. Rice indicated that CDC has been providing data actively to document these concerns and has been calling attention to the urgency of addressing the needs of the ASD community for years. She continued by stating that the workshop was an effort to broaden the conversation and share ideas on how CDC and others can all learn from other fields and improve collaboration to better understand ASD trends.

Analyses of ADDM Network Data Related to: Parental Age, Age at Autism Identification, and Socioeconomic Inequalities in the Prevalence of ASD in the U.S.

M. Durkin

This presentation summarized some analyses of data from CDC's Autism and Developmental Disabilities Monitoring (ADDM) Network related to parental age, age of autism identification, and socioeconomic

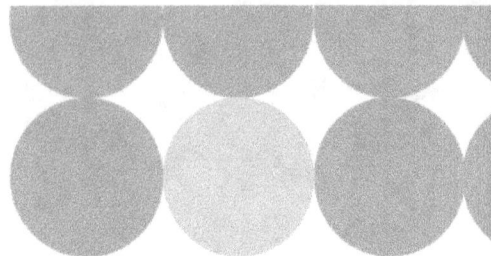

status. A major strength of ADDM Network data on ASD prevalence is that a sizeable proportion (27%) of children identified with ASDs for surveillance did not have a documented ASD classification. This allows us to investigate factors associated with having a previous ASD diagnosis and receiving services for ASD as distinct from having ASD, and to evaluate whether associations are due to differences in ASD risk or to disparities in identification. A consistent finding in recent epidemiologic studies is a positive association between both maternal and paternal age and risk of ASD in offspring. Despite this association and the increasing trend in mean parental age in recent decades, only a very small (less than .5%) proportion of the recent increase in ASD prevalence can be attributed to the increasing age of parents. ASD differs from developmental disabilities overall in its positive association with higher socioeconomic status (SES). Examining SES among Wisconsin ADDM Network data, it was found that the ASD prevalence increased with increasing SES. However, is this due to increased risk or identification disparities? For example, do educated parents have a disproportionate influence on autism awareness or does the risk of autism increase with a higher socioeconomic status? Is a knowledgeable and determined parent of a child with autism more likely to obtain an informed diagnosis? This is likely to be the case, and there is also the potential role of clinician bias and the possible evidence of disparity in access to care. ASD prevalence estimates likely underestimate prevalence in lower SES groups, which implies that we are still underestimating ASD prevalence and can expect some increases if disparity gaps are closed over time. But the fact that we saw a positive association between socioeconomic status and ASD risk in both those with and those without a previous ASD diagnosis suggests that the association might not be entirely due to under-ascertainment of ASD in economically disadvantaged groups.

Panel member discussion:

Panel members raised the question of whether birth order and the effects of stoppage (a family deciding not to have another child after having a child with a disability) have been studied, and if plans are under way to study miscarriages and autism risk. Dr. Durkin indicated that the effect of birth order combined with parental age and sex appear to be additive. The role of stoppage and pregnancy loss cannot be directly or adequately investigated using ADDM data but require longitudinal, birth cohort studies. CDC's Study to Explore Early Development (SEED) will examine prenatal and perinatal risk factors, such as miscarriages. Studying these factors is important because past adverse pregnancy outcomes are understudied. The importance of examining characteristics (such as parental age, and SES) across cohorts to look at changes among subgroups will be important in understanding potential identification and risk factors contributing to ASD prevalence increases.

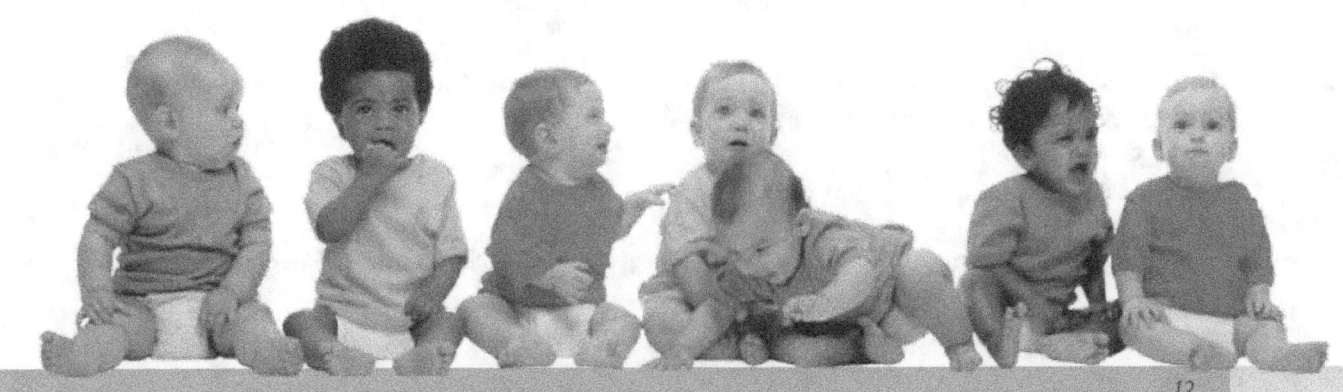

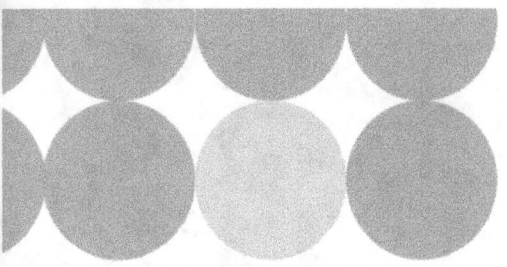

ASD Trends:
U.S. Service-Based Datasets

U.S. Special Education Data
P. Shattuck

This presentation provided an overview of U.S. Department of Education data related to documenting the presence of ASDs among special education students. U.S. Department of Education's Special Education Child Count data is an annual count of children enrolled in special education services. It is an accountability measure required by the Individuals with Disabilities Education Act (IDEA) to show nonexclusion of children with a disability based on select eligibility categories for each state. Autism was not initially a category within the child count dataset, but was added in 1990 with statesreporting to the U.S. Department of Education in 1991. The number of children classified as having autism and receiving special education services has increased since the early 1990s. However, the number is still fewer than would be expected given current prevalence estimates. A special education label is only mildly sensitive, but highly specific, and enrollment counts might not have provided a true prevalence of ASD. Child Count data vary by area and race or ethnicity. The special education system never was intended to serve a public health surveillance role. Thus, several important questions have been raised that focus on (1) understanding how state-level special education criteria for ASDs vary, (2) exploring referral pathways that lead to identification, (3) examining barriers to timely identification, and (4) developing more effective partnerships with the education sector to maximize data sharing. This will lead to a better understanding of the social, economic, and political factors that influence ASD identification in the community and that might contribute to the rise in identification ASDs in prevalence estimates.

Panel member discussion:

Panel members asked how to integrate ASD screening in schools. Dr. Shattuck indicated that a school equivalent of CDC's Learn the Signs. Act Early. program is needed to increase awareness among educators of the signs of ASDs, and should be followed up with a systematic screening protocol to identify children with an ASD. This is important because, until everyone in the schools uses the same criteria, it will be difficult to rely on the validity of the Child Count data for monitoring changes in the actual prevalence of ASDs. Dr. Shattuck also indicated the need for legislative support to allow education and public health to form effective partnerships; often, school systems do not see the value in the Child Count data from a public health perspective. Especially now, schools are working to meet the service needs of the students rather than addressing broader public health issues such as identifying all children with an ASD in the population.

California Department of Developmental Services Data I
I. Hertz-Picciotto

This presentation provided an overview of some ways the California Department of Developmental Services (CA DDS) administrative data have been used to evaluate trends among children receiving services for ASD. Whether due to an artifact or a true increase, ASD prevalence has been high and there is a need to identify the causes. In addition, there already is enough evidence to suggest the importance of environmental causes. There are three main measures of occurrence of a condition: prevalence (the number of cases divided by the number of people in the population at a given time), incidence (the number of new cases among a given population in a defined time divided by the amount of person-time observed during the same period), and cumulative incidence (the number of new cases identified in an extended time period [e.g., from birth] divided by the size of the population without the disorder at the start of the time period). All measures are affected by changes in identification patterns and diagnostic practices. Prevalence data are most useful for service planning and incidence data are useful for etiology. However, a condition where the diagnosis tends to be stable (low mortality rate and it is rare for the diagnosis to change), can result in prevalence and cumulative incidence measures that will be virtually identical over a defined time or age period. For this reason, examining existing data may help us understand ASD trends.

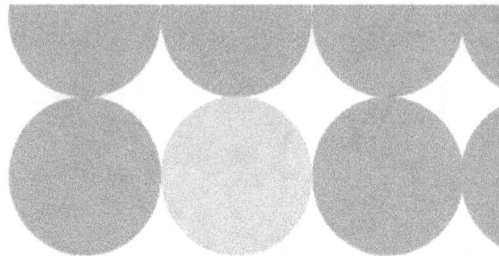

The CA DDS has a statewide database with data from 21 regional centers in the state. The DDS database tracks 5 conditions (autism, epilepsy, cerebral palsy, intellectual disability, and intellectual disability-related conditions). Data collection is passive in that a child must be brought to a CA DDS center and a parent or guardian must request an evaluation to determine if they meet the service provision eligibility criteria. Comparing births in 1990 with those in 2001 (followed to age ten), the cumulative incidence in autism in the CA DDS rose 600%. About 200% of this increase in autism from 1990 through 2001 in the CA DDS database could be explained by trends toward younger age at diagnosis, inclusion of more mild cases, changes in diagnostic criteria, and older ages of mothers. Thus, artifacts related to criteria and methods for ascertainment might explain part but not all of the increase in ASD cumulative incidence in the CA DDS system. To date, there appears to be no leveling off of autism diagnoses, indicating there is considerable likelihood that there has been a true increase in incidence (or risk).

Panel member discussion:

Panel members questioned how the identification artifacts played out across regions. Dr. Hertz-Picciotto indicated that there was substantial variability among the centers (Los Angeles traditionally has had higher ASD rates than other regions of the state). .Each DDS center is run by independent contractors and are managed slightly differently from each other. There also are clusters of ASDs near places where there are well-known treatment centers. A panel member pointed out that it is important to study these identification factors at multiple locations beyond California service data to areas of the U.S. and to also consider international patterns of occurrence.

California Department of Developmental Services Data II

P. Bearman

This presentation summarized additional analyses of data from the CA DDS related to trends in ASD prevalence conducted by Dr. Bearman and colleagues. During the past 30 years, the prevalence of autism has increased dramatically. Examining California birth data from the period 1992 through 2007, there were 8 million births (about 500,000 births per year). Using a sophisticated mapping program of all births and addresses and linking to CA DDS autism data, researchers were able to ascertain parental characteristics, prenatal conditions, and residence during the in utero period and link to data on neighborhoods, socioeconomic status, local toxicants, and other conditions. Examining these data was useful in examining the contribution of diagnostic change to increased prevalence, gaining insight into genetic mechanisms, understanding the spatial structuring or geographic patterns of autism at birth and age of diagnosis, considering diverse individual and community level risk factors, and measuring the potential role of sharing information on autism.

Analysis of the data showed that changes in ASD diagnoses in relation to those for intellectual disability (mental retardation) explained 24% of the increase in autism prevalence in the CA DDS data during the time period analyzed. An analysis was also done to see how administrative data might provide insight into genetic mechanisms. There was a high ASD concordance between identical twins and low concordance between fraternal twins. Over time, there was an increase in ASD among same sex twins and a decrease among opposite sex twins. Another analysis examined the spatial structure (geographic mapping) of the birth residence of children later identified with ASD by DDS. The researchers concluded that ASD birth clusters have been robust over time and do not appear to be due to factors such as education or socioeconomic status. Examining the DDS administrative data has provided insight into risk factors for autism. For example, findings indicated maternal age might be more critical than paternal age; community level characteristics such as geographic spacing are increasingly less salient as ascertainment increases, but still significant; and shorter interpregnancy intervals might confer excess risk. About 50% of ASD prevalence increases in the CA DDS data could be explained by several factors, such as diagnostic change, advancing parental age, social influence of people sharing information on ASDs, and spatial structure. Work is needed to understand what accounts for the other 50%. A project currently is under way to investigate

whether assistive reproductive technology (ART) is related to increased risk of having a child with ASD as identified in CA DDS data by linking with CDC data on births involving ART.

Panel member discussion:

Questions were raised about the autism clusters that were identified using CA DDS data. There was a question as to whether these were true etiologic clusters or if there appeared to be shared identification patterns. Dr. Bearman discussed the idea that clusters might have been due to a shared exposure, such as toxicant, or to a social risk factor. For example, people with children the same age who shared a workplace or social activity might have been more likely to discuss their children and share information about autism, thus leading to increased identification. Or, there might have been reluctance among some groups to reach out to the health care or services system, resulting in decreased identification. A panel member expressed caution about the conclusion of being able to explain about 50% of the increase in DDS ASD prevalence as the approach used to arrive at this estimate was too simplistic and did not take the overlapping relationships between different factors into account. Dr. Bearman relayed his belief that some of the factors operate on different aspects of the spectrum and that the 50% figure was a way of summarizing what is known to date. For example, identification factors, such as shifts in the use of the intellectual disability diagnosis to add autism as another diagnosis or an alternative diagnosis, may operate on the lower end of the spectrum and social influence may operate on the higher end of the spectrum. Factors such as parental age and shorter pregnancy intervals are more likely to be risk factors contributing to ASD increases.

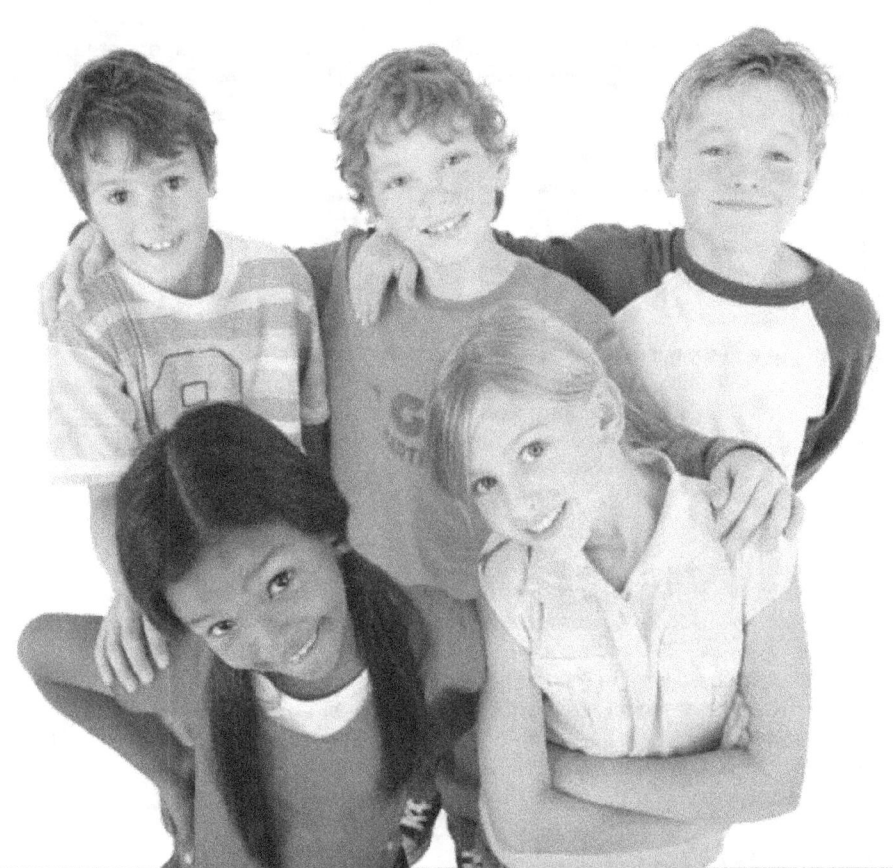

Lessons Learned From Other Conditions and Analytic Methodologies

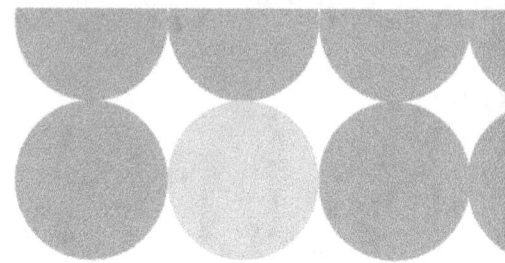

Cancer

R. Etzioni

Changes in cancer trends can be seen from changes in (1) exposures (e.g., smoking, diet, and obesity), (2) diagnosis or detection (e.g., screening and biopsy techniques), and (3) classification (e.g., staging and grading techniques). Dr. Etzioni presented three examples of changes in different types of cancer:

- Lung Cancer—The greatest modifiable risk factor for lung cancer is smoking. The trend line for lung cancer incidence plots has sloped similarly with the trend line for smoking prevalence, meaning the incidence rates of lung cancer have decreased over time (Surveillance, Epidemiology and End Results registry data) as smoking behavior has decreased over time (National Health and Nutrition Examination Survey).

- Colorectal Cancer—Screening rates for colorectal cancer have been increasing over time and the consumption of two or more servings of red meat per week has been decreasing over time. As screening has increased and red meat consumption has decreased, the incidence of colorectal cancer has decreased.

- Prostate Cancer—Prostate-specific antigen (PSA) screening was first introduced in the 1990s, which correlated with the first peak of prostate prevalence. The second prevalence peak occurred when follow-up biopsies became more routine. Researchers attributed the prevalence changes to differences in recording techniques and improvements in grading of cancer (from poorly to moderately to well-differentiated).

Examining patterns of change among a population might explain disease trends due to changes in factors such as the annual frequencies of exposures, availability of screenings, use of new diagnostic technologies, and changes in disease coding. It is important to have data on the occurrence of a condition before and after the change factor being evaluated. It is also helpful if there is a clear change factor that has occurred.

Modeling change is an integral part of cancer surveillance. There are several important lessons learned from this modeling that can be useful when examining changes in ASD prevalence. The basic steps of modeling change are:

- Characterizing changes in disease trends;

- Quantifying changes in the population that might explain trends;

- Identifying a mechanism for the effect of the population trend;

- Estimating the size of the effect on the risk of disease diagnosis; and

- Modeling or simulating experience among the population.

All of these steps are equally necessary and applicable in explaining changes in ASD prevalence. However, modeling techniques might be useful if the potential effects of a factor on prevalence are not known. There is a group called the Cancer Intervention and Surveillance Modeling Network (www.cisnet.cancer.gov) that is working to develop techniques for modeling changes in cancer based on multiple factors. Working with this group might be helpful in understanding ASD prevalence changes.

Parkinson Disease

C. Tanner

Parkinson's disease is a relatively rare disorder that does not have a diagnostic test or definitive marker. Symptoms occur later in life and share some features, such as cognitive decline, with other conditions such as Alzheimer's. The best diagnosis is a face-to-face exam. As with ASDs, population-based surveillance is challenging and there have been changes in diagnostic criteria over time. Also similar to autism, there are questions about the higher prevalence in males and differences by race. One example of examining diagnostic incidence trends of Parkinson's is a study conducted in the Kaiser Permanente Medical Care Program of Northern California (KPMCP). Researchers used active surveillance to examine electronic

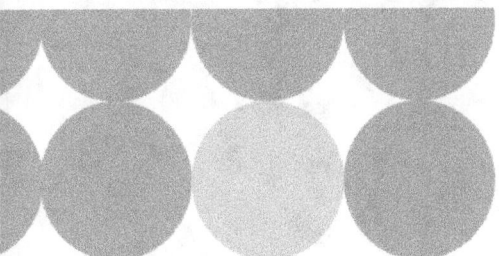

medical records, physician referrals, and computerized databases to identify patients receiving services in community settings. Researchers have identified increased incidence of Parkinson's disease among men and with increasing age, a pattern that has been seen in most populations world-wide. Patterns that were suggested, but not supported by evidence, were higher incidence among Hispanics and the lowest incidence among Blacks. Environmental and genetic risk factors have been associated with Parkinson's disease. At this point, there are few sources of data to examine population trends in Parkinson's disease. The CA Parkinson's Disease Registry is a pilot effort to create a population-based database with active ascertainment and case validation, but is active in only a few counties and no state funds are designated to support the effort. Other efforts at population-based registries have been tried, but in these there is no active mechanism for reporting. Advocacy groups support a national surveillance system for Parkinson's disease, but this has yet to be realized. Researchers are also examining conditions with similar symptoms and/or risk factors to identify common biologic mechanisms. It may be useful to study prevalence changes in other disorders with symptoms that overlap with ASDs and among adults.

Panel member discussion:

A panel member asked if there is a spectrum of conditions similar to ASDs. Dr. Tanner indicated that there are similar clinical syndromes including Parkinsonism. Different disorders have different clinical features and prognoses, but definitive diagnosis is post-mortem.

Asthma
M. King

Asthma is a highly prevalent chronic disease. Studies have shown persistent demographic differences in prevalence, as well as health care use. Asthma surveillance relies on several national datasets to determine prevalence and severity. One of these is the National Health Interview Survey (NHIS). Before 1997, the NHIS measured 12-month prevalence based on self-reports of "having asthma." After 1997, the NHIS measured prevalence by self-report of a "doctor's diagnosis" of asthma and included lifetime, past 12-months, and whether an attack occurred in past 12-months. The current measure of prevalence is similar to the projected 12-month rate, and the prevalence is higher among children than adults with racial differences observed as well. The Behavioral Risk Factor Surveillance System (BRFSS) allows state-specific estimates of asthma and enables CDC to conduct an asthma call-back survey. The BRFSS allows CDC to determine a population-based prevalence, as well as an at-risk–based rate. An at-risk–based rate is the number of affected people within the population having certain risk factors. While asthma prevalence has increased over time, actual asthma attack rates have been relatively stable. The reasons for overall prevalence increases are not known, but there are sociodemographic disparities in identification and service use. Changes in survey measurement have affected asthma estimates.

Panel member discussion:

There was a question about the content of the call-back survey. Dr. King indicated this that this survey provides a chance to find out more about health care needs and use, effects on quality of life, and other information on the functional effect of asthma and service use related to asthma. Another question was about the availability of linking asthma data with environmental factors such as air pollution. Dr. King stated that data are not available to look at direct measures among individuals in the population over time, but different datasets could be linked to conduct ecologic analysis of asthma survey data based on residence and air quality, for example.

Schizophrenia
E. Susser

There are many parallels between schizophrenia and ASDs in the attempts to estimate incidence and historical changes in incidence. With respect to schizophrenia and related psychoses, two landmark

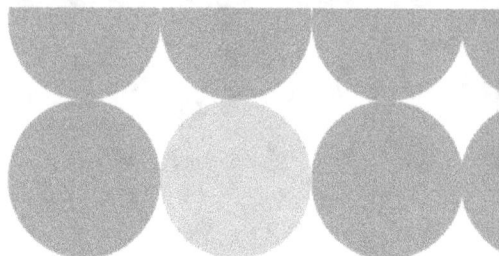

World Health Organization (WHO) studies can be used to mark shifts in thinking about schizophrenia, as well as about how studies of schizophrenia should be conducted. First, the International Pilot Study of Schizophrenia (IPSS), conducted in the 1960s, was designed to determine if schizophrenia was a culturally bound disorder and if it was a "real" disorder (some people hypothesized that schizophrenia was a social construction). The study used standardized criteria in a multinational study and many regions of the world were included. Researchers found schizophrenia in all settings; that finding is still questioned, but is supported by the findings of other types of studies. Second, the WHO "Ten Country Study" examined whether the incidence and course of schizophrenia varied across sociocultural settings. The study also had a novel design for determining incidence. It inaugurated the "first contact" design, now widely used and considered a "gold standard", in which researchers ascertain all people seeking help for a possible psychosis for the first time, within a defined population.

Based on misinterpretation of the results of these (and other) studies, the prevailing summary of schizophrenia from 1980 to about 2005 was that there was a lifetime risk of schizophrenia of 1%, and that this figure remained constant over time and place. The current view on schizophrenia is different; it is clear that the occurrence varies across populations and population subgroups, the clearest example being the very high rates among some immigrants who are ethnic minorities (mainly documented among immigrant groups in the United Kingdom and Netherlands). This variation is not inconsistent with the results of the WHO studies, but is inconsistent with the way these results were interpreted by most schizophrenia researchers and clinicians as showing constant rates overtime (not by the authors themselves, who were cautious in their conclusions). The WHO studies were not designed to examine change over time. Although other studies have attempted to examine change over time (e.g. registry studies), the results have been inconsistent, and the data weak (e.g. due to changes in diagnostic practices and systems). As a result, with the exception of one or two particular locations, we cannot at present draw conclusions as to whether schizophrenia incidence has changed over time. The discrepancy between studies of the course of schizophrenia, and interpretation of those results (again, not by the authors) is even more striking, but I do not have time to elaborate on this during this presentation.

There are several important lessons learned from studies of schizophrenia that could be useful when examining changes in ASD prevalence. For example, with regard to the notion of "constant" incidence over place and time, fixed thinking about schizophrenia was allowed to override the available data. The idea that schizophrenia occurred worldwide and that there was at most a very modest variation in incidence was accepted as true for a long time, and still taught in many psychiatry and other mental health professional training programs. This lesson is relevant to ASDs to help understand how to interpret ASD data. There have been different waves of ideology which have influenced the way in which the data on incidence of ASDs have been interpreted, and in particular, on whether they demonstrate a "true" increase or not ("true" means over and above an increase due to changes in ascertainment and help-seeking). The schizophrenia story helps one to recognize the power of ideology in the interpretation of such data, and the need to be cognizant of it. He noted his personal view is that the data on whether there has been a "true" increase in autism are simply inconclusive, but that the overall evidence favors the position that a part of the increase is "true".

Panel member discussion:

Panel members asked if there was a specific way in which those in the ASD field could learn from the schizophrenia example? Dr. Susser responded that there have been different waves of ideology in how autism and related conditions have been interpreted and people tend to look at data as either, "yes, there has been an increase", or "no, there has not been an increase". It would be really helpful for those working with ASDs to not look through the data using those lenses, but to ask questions openly. Dr. Susser further stated that we do not need to be committed to either position to use data to advocate and to improve services. There was another question on subtypes of schizophrenia. Dr. Susser indicated that subtypes typically have not been reliable over time. Dr. Susser also commented that if a disorder persists

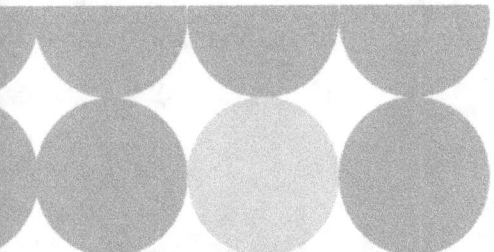

over generations, we also should be consider examining if there are selective mutations occurring or reframing to consider a selective advantage associated with the condition.

Simulation Studies

S. Galea

This presentation provided a brief overview of simulation studies as a method to understand prevalence changes. Changes in ASD prevalence have been and continue to be an observed phenomenon, yet the problem lies in identifying the causes for the changes. Causal models, including sufficient-component cause models, can shed some light on the joint effects of multiple exposures. However, these models are unable to consider timing in a dynamic way or connections between individuals. A possible solution is to use complex systems models. Complex systems approaches are computational approaches that use computer-based algorithms to model dynamic interactions between individuals within and across levels of influence (such as social networks and neighborhoods) using simulated populations. Complex systems models can incorporate multilevel determinants of population health, connections between individuals, and patterns of feedback between exposures and outcomes over time.

An example of trying to understand health problems seen after disasters was presented using a type of analytic strategy called "agent-based modeling" to predict changes among heterogeneous populations. The goal was to model outcomes observed by varying the variables that might have contributed to the observed pattern. There could have been several different sets of variables that produced the same outcome. A lesson that might be important when examining reasons for ASD trends is that complex systems models point to different possible explanations for observed phenomenon. However, they can be used in conjunction with empirical data to narrow down possible explanations and can play a central role in epidemiological analyses.

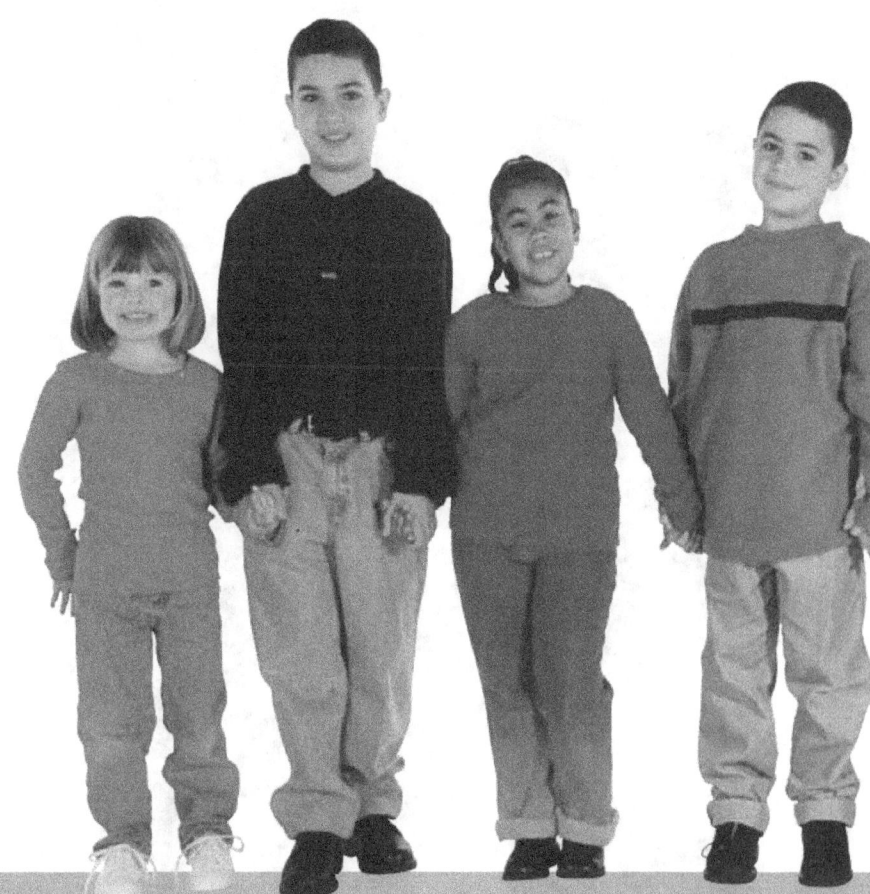

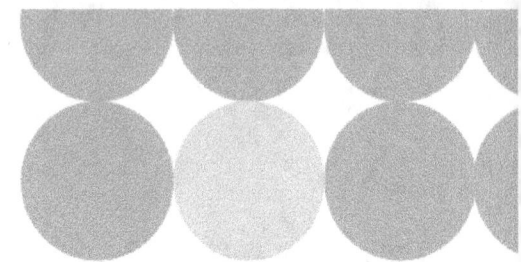

Open Comments

The workshop included presentations and discussions among panel members. However, the meeting was open to anyone to register and attend in person or via webinar. Nonpanel members were able to provide written comments before and after the workshop, as well oral statements during an open period of the workshop. Comments included concern about increases in ASDs, the need to find out what has changed in our environment, the larger than expected number of children and young adults with an ASD, and the cost to society. Many of the public comments focused on concern about the role of vaccines in autism, with disappointment expressed about the lack of research on vaccine safety. In particular, studies of vaccinated and unvaccinated children and mitochondrial disease were requested. In addition, concerns were raised about the cumulative effect of the vaccine schedule and vaccine ingredients, as well as the need to consider a child's immune status prior to giving vaccinations. Suggestions were made for other studies such as of young children's development from birth to 2 years of age and to determine if there are specific subgroups of children with ASDs, such as those with gastrointestinal sensitivities. A man with an ASD expressed the belief that it is possible to be successful with an ASD and offered himself as an example of someone who once relied on public assistance, but is now successfully employed and lives independently. He also expressed gratitude for CDC's work in vaccine safety and satisfaction with receiving vaccines to protect from known diseases. Other comments included frustration with the delays parents face in getting a diagnosis of autism, despite bringing concerns to the attention of professionals. Other comments included concern about non-scientific expertise among panelists and interest in the latest research findings and plans for future research related to ASDs. Workshop organizers, panelists, and stakeholders were asked to consider these comments when discussing priorities for evaluating changes in ASD prevalence.

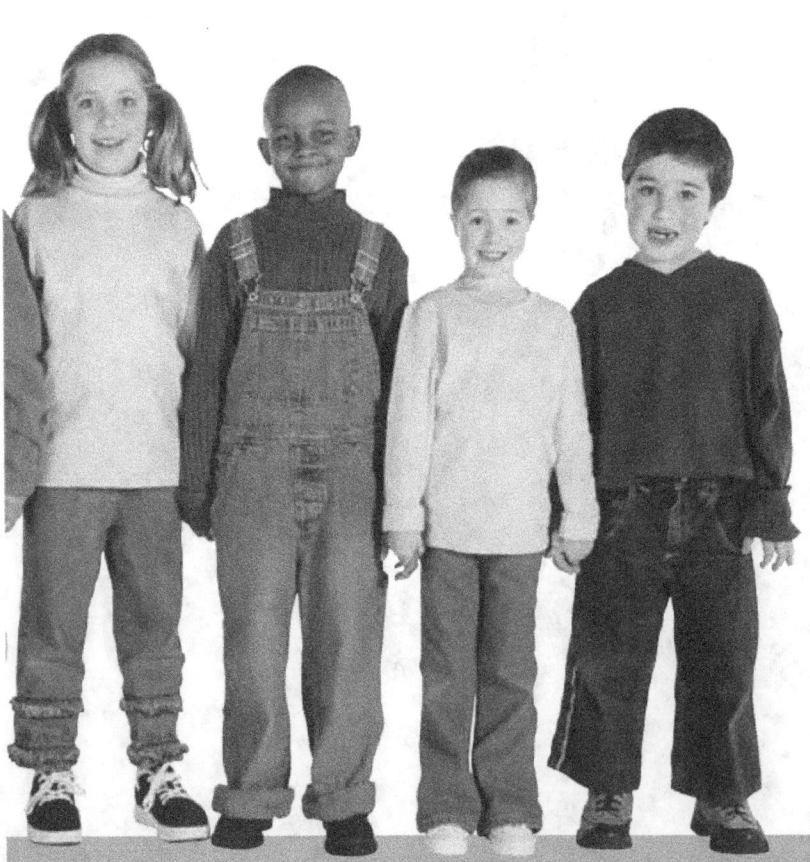

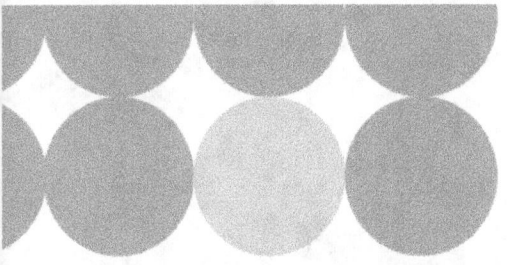

Panel Session Summaries

The workshop featured four breakout panel discussions, with each panel asked to discuss questions related to ASD prevalence. The panelists' discussion, ideas, and suggestions were compiled by the panel chairs. Panel members consisted of epidemiologists and scientists with experience in epidemiology and surveillance of autism or other complex conditions and community stakeholders (representatives from autism organizations, parents of children with an ASD, and adults with an ASD). Following is a summary of the panel discussions and their ideas for addressing questions related to ASD prevalence trends.

Panel 1: Utility of ASD Prevalence Data

Panel Chair: *A. Singer*
Panelists: *C. Cunniff, W. Zahorodny, R. Kirby, M. Lopez, R. Grinker, D. Mandell*, L. Grossman*, W. Dunaway, M. Rosanoff, J. Zimmerman, B. Mulvihill, J. Charles*

*Invited participant unable to attend remotely or in-person at last minute due to unforeseen circumstances.

The discussion and questions addressed by Panel 1 focused on how ASD prevalence data are used in the community by different stakeholders and sought to identify ways in which data collection and reporting on the population prevalence and characteristics of people with an ASD could be further developed.

Q1. What does having ASD prevalence information do for stakeholders (parents, professionals, people with an ASD, researchers, scientists, policy makers, service providers)?

The panelists indicated that ASD prevalence data are used to:

- Empower the community, confirming what parents and educators experience
- Drive public policy
- Support the need for service provisions and development
- Support the need for professional development and systems planning
- Support the need for additional research

At the community level, prevalence data have informed stakeholders about needed improvements in identifying people with an ASD and helped direct research which may ultimately lead to information about etiology. Similarly, the resulting increase in ASD awareness and knowledge among parents, care-givers, and communities has increased the quality of social and behavioral descriptions by clinicians and service providers when a child has been referred for an evaluation. This has resulted in parents being more equipped to discuss concerns with professionals. Clinicians have found that having ASD prevalence information increases awareness of the need to identify children and facilitates having a conversation with parents about concerns. It also has provided information to help clinicians advocate for needed resources for identification, referral, and intervention. Researchers have used prevalence data as justification for etiologic and intervention research, and the increased awareness of ASD has increased their own career choices to be engaged in meaningful work. Individuals with an ASD have also benefitted from ASD prevalence data. Increased ASD awareness has resulted in positive community connections and increased information has allowed them to help themselves and others understand their experience.

Prevalence data also have empowered communities by confirming what parents and educators have been experiencing and providing evidence for robust advocacy. ASD prevalence estimates have provided a starting point to assess service and support needs for individuals, families, and communities. On a policy level, awareness of the Autism and Developmental Disabilities Monitoring (ADDM) Network has allowed scientists and researchers, in some states, easier access to data sources and records for surveillance purposes, thus increasing the accuracy of ASD estimates. Prevalence estimates also have informed policy efforts to create an infrastructure to support children with an ASD (e.g., child care, intervention, education, transition services); understand and address lifespan issues (e.g, housing training, employment, health

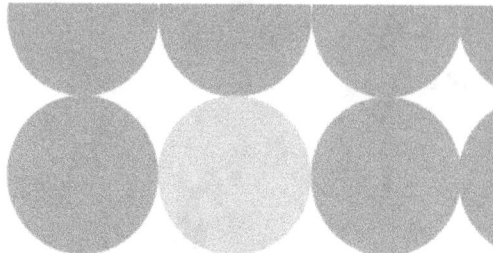

and wellness); drive public policy and programs (e.g., insurance coverage and health care legislation); and support the need for service deployment, systems planning, and additional research funding.

Q2. How are stakeholders actually using ASD prevalence information?

ASD prevalence data are included at the beginning of many, if not most, research publications and grant applications related to ASDs because they provide an estimate of the population-level effect of the conditions. In particular, recent estimates indicating that ASDs are more common than previously thought have motivated the need to better understand the course, causes, and supports related to ASDs. In addition to putting the scope of need into perspective, recent ASD prevalence estimates have prompted some states to pass mandatory reporting laws, establish autism task force groups or autism councils, pass legislation affecting service provision, or offer grants to school districts for supplemental funding related to autism. Examples of how states have used ASD prevalence data follow:

- South Carolina used prevalence data to show the need for improving access to services when drafting and passing insurance reform.
- New Jersey passed laws related to ASDs and mandatory reporting, compelling insurance companies to provide services and providing additional grants to schools.
- Alabama appointed an autism coordinator for the state based on the effects of the prevalence data.

Q3. What types of ASD prevalence information and descriptions of the population are useful to stakeholders?

For individuals, families, and communities, having ASD prevalence data that are applicable to more specific local areas and states can better inform advocacy and service planning efforts. ASD prevalence data are population-based and are not easily applicable at the individual level. In addition to understanding the population effects of ASDs, families and communities continue to seek ways of making the information more relevant for their individual circumstances. Specific recommendations included:

- Improving communication with the community (e.g., families, individuals with an ASD, professionals, policy makers, and researchers) to help put the prevalence data into context.
- Providing more in-depth information on what an ASD diagnosis means for an individual across his or her lifespan, and what support systems such an individual needs or will need.
- Collecting and reporting data on functional level and effects of ASD, subtypes, developmental characteristics, and associated conditions (in addition to overall ASD prevalence estimates).

Q4. What questions do stakeholders expect epidemiology and prevalence studies, in particular, to answer?

The panel noted that community stakeholders want the data to be useful at the community and individual levels. At the community level, ASD prevalence estimates can inform larger needs (identification, supports, policy, and research). For the individual person, as suggested in Q3's discussion, more detailed data on functioning and characteristics would be helpful. Prevalence numbers should inform preparation for the needs of a growing population. In addition to describing the population, prevalence studies could provide a baseline for evaluating interventions and gauging service needs. Some panel members called for more data on the link between prevalence and etiology. For example, would lower prevalence in some areas or subgroups indicate potential protective mechanisms? Prevalence studies should be accompanied by data collection on specific symptoms or biological measures, interventions, and trajectories over time.

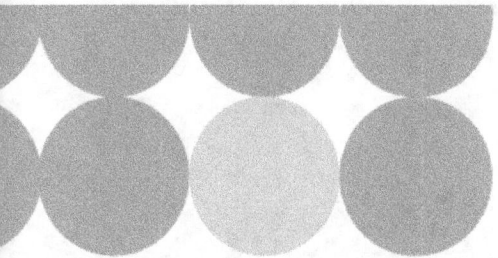

Panel 2: U.S.-Based ASD Service Data

Panel Chair: *L. Croen*

Panelists: *P. Shattuck, P. Bearman, M. Kogan, S. Visser, I. Hertz-Piciotto, L. Miller, A. Bakian, K. Van Naarden Braun, L. Lee, T. Baroud, P. Bell, R. Etzioni, Y. Kim*

Panel 2 discussed databases that exist to serve the administrative functions of tracking service use, or were developed for specific studies. Although not designed to identify all children with an ASD among the population, these databases might serve as useful tools for looking at trends in identification, characteristics, and service use that will help explain population-based ASD prevalence trends. Some of the databases or datasets noted that could be explored for examining administrative or reported prevalence issues include:

All-Payer Claims Database (APCD; combines outpatient data from all claims databases)

California Department of Developmental Services (CA DDS) database

Department of Education/Individuals with Disabilities Education Act (IDEA) Child Count (also, Special Education Longitudinal Study)

Hospital Discharge Data

Interactive Autism Network (IAN) survey

Kaiser Permanente® membership databases

Centers for Medicaid and Medicare Services (CMS)

National Health Interview Survey (NHIS)

National Survey of Children's Health (NSCH)

National Survey of Children with Special Health Care Needs (NSCSHCN)

State registries (New Jersey, Utah, West Virginia)

Vaccine Adverse Event Reporting System (VAERS)

Q1. What are the top three immediate (within 1 to 2 years) priority analyses needed to understand ASD trends using existing U.S.-based datasets?

Panelists discussed several analyses that could be pursued, including:

- Conducting a life-course study of ASD identification, service use, and characteristics. Tracking life history can help determine if the ways people come into the system are changing. Researchers could examine first concerns and average age at first diagnosis, and what happens before and after an ASD diagnosis occurs among those in successive birth cohorts. Kaiser Permanente® membership data could be used to explore this.

- Examining trends in comorbidities among children with ASDs over time and trends in the use of treatments among parents over time. For example, a potential research question might include "Does survivorship of a mental or physical illness by parents (e.g., bipolar disorder) affect the trend in ASD prevalence among children? Kaiser Permanente® membership data or perhaps Medicaid data could be used to explore this type of question.

- Examining behavioral screening data to investigate trends in ASD diagnosis over time. Potential data sources could include the ADDM Network, as well as research programs, insurer databases, and primary care practices that have administered developmental screening tests over time.

- Examining trends in other behaviorally defined conditions (e.g., attention-deficit/hyperactivity disorder, depression, and anxiety) in U.S. population-based datasets (e.g., the National Survey of Children's Health). This could be addressed by ADDM Network data (among children with an ASD).

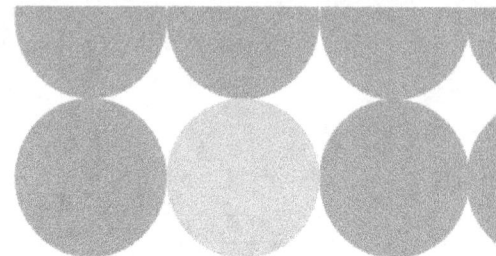

- Looking at ASD prevalence trends over time among different immigrant groups. This might inform trends and prevalence rates in terms of eliminating certain risk factors. However, it is difficult to disentangle if observed rates are lower among immigrants either because of immigrants' lack of familiarity with the U.S. health care system U.S. (including how it operates), or because of reluctance on the part of immigrants to seek medical attention for developmental disorders, or both.

- Further examining the respondents to national surveys who had at least one child ever diagnosed with an ASD and who reported the child no longer had an ASD diagnosis at the time of the survey There is a need to understand why some children may have been reported to have an ASD at one time, but not at the time of the survey.

Q2. What are the top three next (within 3 to 5 year) priority analyses needed to understand ASD trends using existing U.S.-based datasets?

Panelists discussed several potential analyses, including:

- Conducting multilevel modeling with Special Education Child Count or other datasets. Enhanced analysis might help answer questions regarding administrative prevalence trends in schools and communities.

- Using Special Education Child Count data from both IDEA Part C Early Intervention for 0-3 year-olds and IDEA Part B for 3-21 year-olds to track identification, services, and developmental trajectories at the individual level.

- Linking all-payer claims databases with state autism registries to track ASD diagnostic or billing codes, along with additional billing and pharmaceutical claims, to provide information concerning comorbid conditions.

- Taking simulation-based approaches to data analysis, and evaluating the models using real data from epidemiologic studies.

- Using Medicaid data to examine trends over time in ASD and related diagnoses among those receiving Medicaid services. Also, evaluate children longitudinally to examine changes in diagnoses and services.

- Collaborating with the National Institute of Mental Health (NIMH) to better understand the factors associated with the persistence of parent-reported ASD diagnosis. (NIMH has partnered with the Health Resources and Services Administration and the Centers for Disease Control and Prevention, and currently is conducting a follow-up study of the NSCSHCN for families of children who were reported ever to have had a diagnosis of an ASD.)

Q3. Can the existing data systems be enhanced (e.g., adding analyses, data collection) to better answer questions about the changing ASD prevalence? If not, why not and what else is needed?

Panelists discussed several enhancements, including:

- Enhancing use of Child Count Special Education Data by
    » Documenting state differences in identifying children as eligible for autism special education services and documenting the methodology for obtaining and reporting these data to make better sense of special education data.
    » Conducting studies to evaluate how children with autism are identified at schools.
    » Enabling individual-level child data to be accessed for study purposes and pooled together.

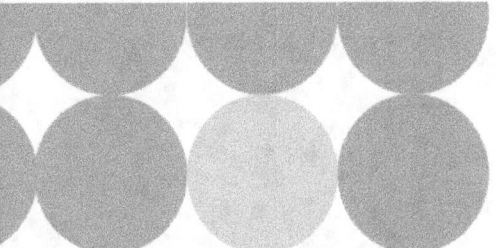

- Enhancing use of surveys by
  - » Conducting needed validation studies of parent-reported data.
  - » Exploring whether national surveys (e.g., National Immunization Survey, NHIS, NSCH, VAERS) could be used to examine ASDs among vaccinated versus unvaccinated groups.
  - » Using national surveys to examine service use and needs.
  - » Adding questions to the IAN Survey to assess beliefs about causes of ASDs.
- Enhancing data access and coordination by
  - » Partnering with analytic powerhouses (e.g., Google) to develop new strategies to take advantage of the huge amounts of data that will become available in upcoming years (e.g., data enhancements from health care reform and electronic health records). This will require public and private partnerships.
  - » Making ASDs reportable conditions in more states. However, it was noted that making a condition reportable does not improve the ability to understand trends, but it is a useful method to establish public health authority to collect additional data to track trends.
  - » Collaborating with the National Environmental Public Health Tracking Network (EPHTN) to potentially access environmental risk factor and other environmental public health tracking data at the population-level.
- Creating new data collections for
  - » Using qualitative methods to understand pathways to screening and diagnosis.
  - » Monitoring trends in ASD prevalence prospectively to rule out "artificial" factors. Consistently conduct developmental and ASD screening at given ages with diagnostic follow-up and documentation of each step and outcomes.
  - » Developing methods to track the effects of information dissemination across parent networks via the Internet or other social media.

Panel 3: Autism and Developmental Disabilities (ADDM) Network Data

Panel Chair: *G. Dawson*
Panelists: *S. Galea, G. McGwin, O. Devine, A. Correa, M. Zack, P. Yoon, M. Maenner, J. Daniels, L. Schieve, S. Pettygrove, M. Wingate, J. E. Robison, P. C. Marvin*

The questions and discussion of Panel 3 focused on identifying immediate, next, and future priorities for enhancing the data collection, analysis, and reporting of ASD prevalence and descriptive data by the ADDM Network to betterunderstand trends.

Q1. What are the top three immediate (next 1 to 2 years) priority analyses needed to understand ASD trends using existing ADDM Network data?

Panelists discussed the following priorities:

- Conducting simulation studies to predict the anticipated course of ASD prevalence, informed by existing ADDM Network data, by
  - » Identifying and using more complex, nuanced modeling approaches to simultaneously examine multiple identification (intrinsic and extrinsic) and risk factors across cohorts (this will be challenging because several factors are confounded).
  - » Using ADDM Network data to inform assumptions in simulation models of ASD prevalence trends.

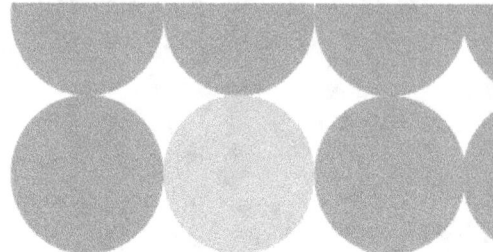

- Conducting analyses that will help explain variations in ASD prevalence across geography and subgroups by

  » Providing information about risk factors related to parental age.

  » Examining data on ASD prevalence for disparities in identification to inform diagnostic and access to service needs.

  » Comparing changes in ASD prevalence among children with more a narrowly defined autistic disorder diagnosis to with those with a broader ASD diagnosis, as autistic disorder might be less influenced by increased public awareness.

- Using methods to maximize the number of children with an ASD in the population identified by the ADDM Network by

  » Performing additional validation studies including direct screening and assessment at other ADDM Network sites and using the results to enhance estimates of ASD prevalence. [Note that a validation study in the Atlanta site (Avchen et al., 2010) found that the records-based approach had good specificity but low sensitivity indicating that ADDM Network ASD case classifications are consistent with clinical examination, but that some children with ASDs are not identified using current methods. Therefore, ADDM Network prevalence estimates likely underestimate ASD prevalence.]

Q2. What are the top three (within 3 to 5 years) priority analyses needed to understand ASD trends using existing ADDM Network data?

Panelists discussed the following potential next priorities:

- Conducting analyses to better understand ASD prevalence trends and current and future needs of adolescents and adults with an ASD by

  » Examining an older cohort to better understand the changes in prevalence over time. This could be done by

    * Surveying a previously-characterized cohort of 8-year-olds when they are older to determine if prevalence estimates are the same in this cohort at older ages.

  » Identifying methods for estimating lifetime prevalence and characterizing developmental trajectories by

    * Examining how ASD symptom presentation may change across cohorts and individuals across the lifespan.

    * Identifying methods to examine the effects of early intervention and whether changing symptom profiles may have on ASD prevalence estimates.

  » Conducting studies of ASD prevalence among adults by

    * Identifying appropriate methods for characterizing ASD prevalence at different ages.

    * Addressing the ethical concerns of identifying adults with an ASD who may not want that classification.

    * Characterizing outcomes and service and support needs.

  » Using ADDM Network data to better understand risk factors for ASDs by

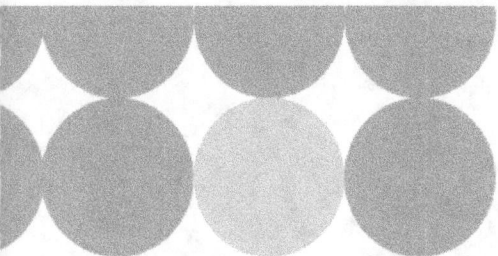

* Recognizing that ADDM Network data might not be well-designed to examine risk factors at the individual level; however, use the data to characterize whether some risk factors have changed among the population and correlate to ASD prevalence changes.

Q3. Can the ADDM Network be enhanced to better answer questions about changing ASD prevalence? If yes, how? If no, why not and what else is needed?

Panelists discussed building on the existing ADDM Network infrastructure by

- Developing ways of better capturing the heterogeneity and complexity of ASD phenotypes.

- Expanding ADDM Network dataset linkages to other datasets (e.g., health, education, service, environmental data) to enrich data completeness and use for examining risk factors.

- Collecting follow-up data on cohorts studied previously at later ages to better understand trends over time and outcomes.

- Collecting more extensive data as part of ongoing surveillance using additional methods such as direct screening and diagnostic confirmation to obtain the most complete estimates of ASD prevalence in the U.S.

Panel 4 –What Else Is Needed To Understand ASD Trends?

Panel Chair: *M. Durkin*
Panelists: *K. Crider, E. Susser, C. Lawler, C. Tanner, M. King, S. Shapira, D. Schendel, J. Nicholas, W. McMahon, J. Constantino, C. Newschaffer, L. Perner, M. Blaxill, E. London, G. Windham, K. Merikangas*

Panel 4 engaged in an open discussion on some of the "big picture" issues related to understanding ASD trends, including whether it is possible to fully understand reasons for ASD prevalence increases, ways to move forward with collaborations and new methods, and what else could be done to improve the understanding of ASD trends.

Q1. Can the question of the relative contribution of identification or risk factors, or both, on ASD prevalence during the last 20 years be answered? If not, why not? If yes, what are the three primary questions that need to be addressed by epidemiology?

Panel members offered a range of perspectives on whether it will ever be possible to understand the relative contributions of identification and risk in increasing ASD prevalence. There was agreement that the ASD prevalence is a huge public health problem and that many individuals and families are affected globally. Panel members did not agree about whether it was possible ever to understand fully all the reasons behind increasing ASD prevalence. One panelist asserted that the question already has been answered: Of course there has been an increase because there has an increase in the number of cases and autism is an epidemic and needs to be treated as a public health emergency. Others noted that autism is a disorder of social behavior and that trends over time in its frequency are affected by corresponding changes in social context, perceptions, awareness, knowledge, diagnostic practices, and availability of services. However, there was a general sense that it is possible to move forward and to be more specific in documenting potential reasons for ASD prevalence trends. Several challenges were mentioned, such as insurmountable measurement error, overlap and confounding of multiple identification and risk factors, and poorly defined subtypes with limited information on biological underpinnings to explain phenotypes. It is unlikely that prevalence trend data will explain the etiology of a complex set of conditions, such as ASDs, but these data can identify clues for further mechanistic studies (e.g., increased risk by sex, geography, and birth characteristics). By better understanding what causes autism, maybe we can understand the

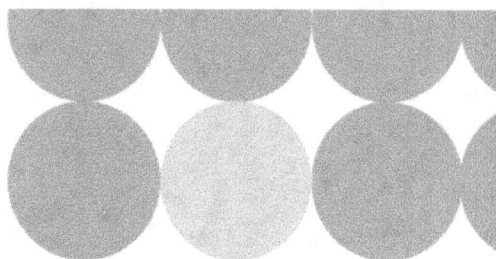

increases in measured prevalence. In addition, panelists noted that we need more clarity on phenotypes, expression across the lifespan, and trends in other conditions. Others thought that, although we might not be able to use prevalence data to make discoveries about how to prevent or cure ASDs, we can use prevalence data to assess needs and improve the lives of those affected by ASDs. This could lead to a focus on services and figuring out how to improve identification and access to such services.

Q2. How can efforts to understand ASD trends be informed by other fields or conditions (e.g., comparison with other conditions, sharing methodology, analytic techniques, etc.)? How can that best be accomplished?

Panelists discussed several potential collaborations, including:

- Comparing ASD prevalence trends to trends in other neurodevelopmental disorders.

- Collaborating with scientists investigating epigenetic effects in cancer and other fields to better understand gene–environment interactions in neurodevelopment.

- Examining subgroups of children with an ASD (e.g., children with fragile X syndrome and ASD) to determine if there are specific risk factors that can be identified among these children with increased risk for developing ASD.

- Analyzing new bioinformatics and computational tools and approaches to better understand complicated systems and interactions.

- Conducting translational research because existing ASD criteria are not mapped to biology and etiology. Translational investigators could help bridge the gap between diagnostic criteria and biology.

Q3. What else is needed to understand reasons for trends?

During the discussions for Questions 1 and 2, several propositions were made for better understanding ASD prevalence trends, including:

- Seeking public–private partnerships to support data collection, analyses, and usage of data.

- Providing funding opportunities to encourage use of existing datasets.

- Expanding use of analytic techniques for examining population trend data by
    - » Using modeling approaches to supplement observed data.
    - » Comparing multiple identification and risk factors that might contribute to prevalence changes.

- Expanding ASD prevalence efforts to include very young children and adults.

- Understanding patterns in ASD prevalence among subgroups (e.g., subtypes, males and females, geographic variation, comorbidities) to evaluate whether changes likely are due to identification or risk factors:

- Expanding the methodology for looking at ASD prevalence by
    - » Developing methods to conduct cross-sectional studies across successive birth cohorts that simultaneously ascertain parent-reported descriptions of developmental characteristics, intellectual functioning, ASD and comorbid symptoms, research diagnosis (categorical or observational), community diagnoses, and family characteristics (sibling recurrence).

- Understanding and improving ASD identification by
    - » Measuring ASDs dimensionally and quantifying the traits that make up the ASDs.

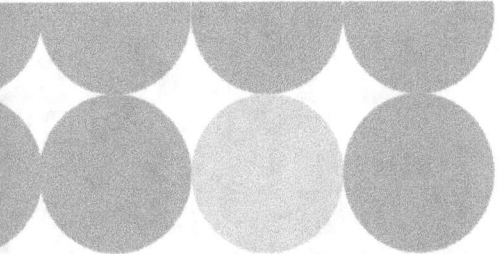

» Measuring any overlap with other conditions and typical development, determining if is there a continuum of symptoms.

» Improving tools for culturally sensitive screening and case confirmation among large populations.

» Developing methods for measuring disability and monitoring functional limitations in individuals with ASD.

» Using data on identification of ASDs to identify gaps and improve community practice.

· Improving community engagement and communication between individuals and families affected by autism, professionals providing services for people with autism, researchers, and policy makers by

» Fostering broader understanding of the strengths and challenges associated with ASDs so people with ASDs have access to the community.

» Utilizing ASD prevalence estimates to develop programs and practices that support the positive development of people with ASDs.

» Realizing that autism is not an academic issue for the many individuals and families affected by ASD, and listening to the concerns of parents of children and individuals with an ASD.

» Sharing information with leadership and policy makers to respond to this health crisis.

· Making sure public health is part of the Interagency Autism Coordinating Committee (IACC) Strategic Plan and input is sought from a range of stakeholders via annual research plan updates.

· Noting that, while trends are important, understanding them might require a better understanding of the etiology and heterogeneity of autism, as well as changes over time in diagnostic practices. These goals can be achieved by

» Advancing basic science on biologic and environmental mechanisms.

» Increasing the types of study methods used in research and service studies such as

* Conducting prospective studies that examine biology, phenotypes, identification patterns, and service needs and use.

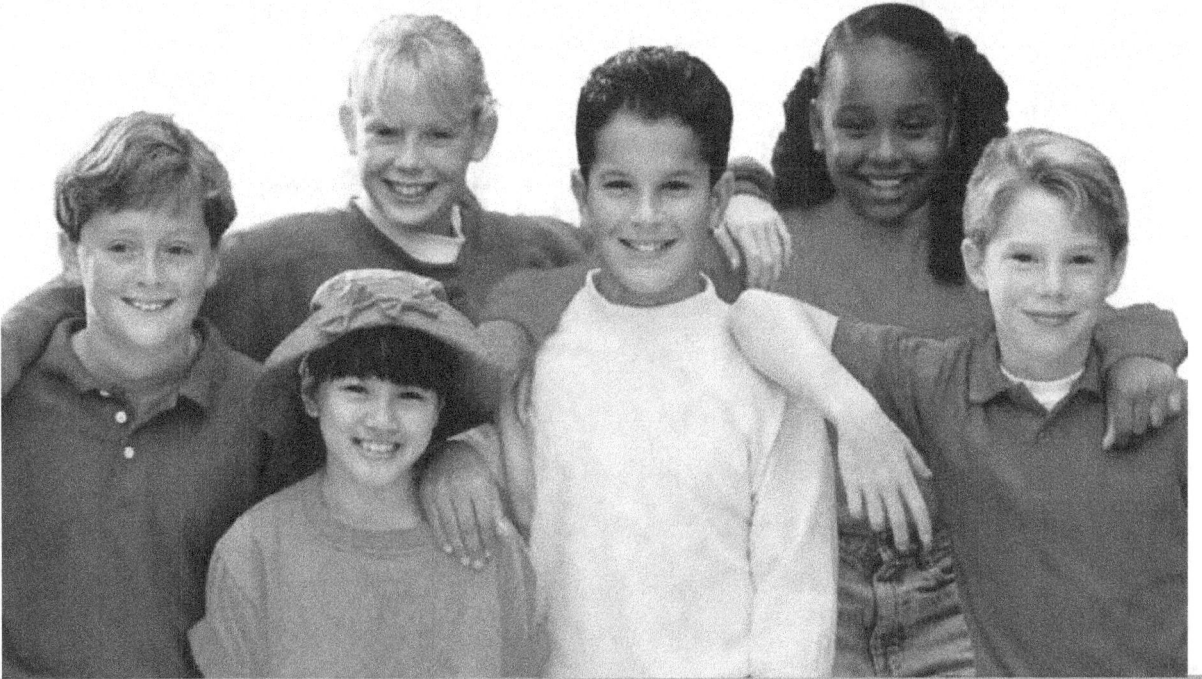

Appendix A: Workshop Agenda

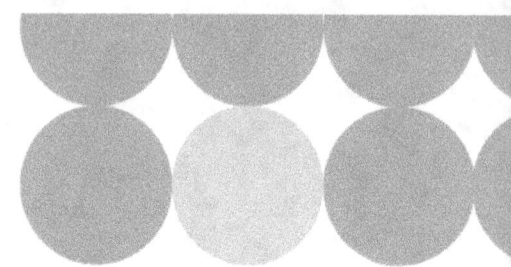

Workshop on U.S. Data to Evaluate Changes in the Prevalence
of the Autism Spectrum Disorders (ASDs)

**Co-Sponsored by the National Center on Birth Defects and Developmental Disabilities,
Centers for Disease Control and Prevention (CDC) and Autism Speaks**

Tuesday, February 1, 2011
Location: Centers for Disease Control and Prevention,
Tom Harkin Global Communications Center, 1600 Clifton Road, N.E., Atlanta, Georgia
Building 19, Auditorium B1/B2

7:30–8:00 .... Check-in

8:00–8:05 .... Welcome — *C. Boyle and G. Dawson*

8:05–10:00 .... Background and purpose

- What do we know about ASD prevalence? — *M. Yeargin-Allsopp*

  » General summary of ASD prevalence

- Framework for this meeting — *C. Rice*

  » What might be influencing temporal patterns in prevalence?

    * Intrinsic Identification – methodology/measurement

    * Extrinsic Identification - (awareness and classification)

    * Risk – (multiple biologic and environmental)

  » Questions to address (For U.S. service data, ADDM, and the field, more generally)

    * What we can do now? (analysis with existing data)

    * What should we do next? (building on existing data systems)

    * What else is needed? (analyses, data collection, others)

- 8:30–8:45 .... A mode for assessing the contribution of various risk factors to recent ASD prevalence increase in the U.S. — *L. Schieve*

  » Examples using selected prenatal and perinatal risk factors.

- 8:45–9:00 .... ASD genetic variation and gene-environment interaction — K. Crider

- 9:00–9:45 .... Examples of analyses in progress from the Autism and Developmental Disabilities Monitoring (ADDM) Network

  » ADDM Network Overview — C. Rice

  » Changes in ASD diagnostic criteria

  » Parental age, dx age, SES — M. Durkin

    * Hypothesis

    * Methods

    * Findings

    * What else could be done to understand ASD trends using this dataset?

    * What else could be done to understand ASD trends?

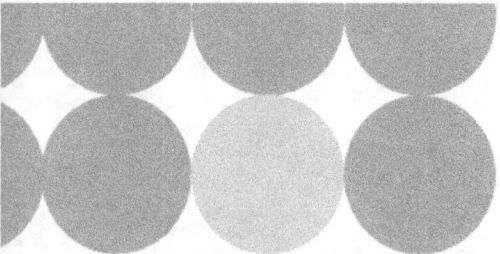

10:00–10:50 ....ASD Trends: U.S. single source datasets (ED and CA DDS data)

- U.S. Special Education Data — P. Shattuck

- CA DDS Data — I. Hertz-Picciotto, P. Bearman

  » Brief overview of evidence of prevalence changes.
  » What factors contribute to the change in prevalence over time? (is it possible to distinguish the relative contribution of various intrinsic identification, extrinsic identification, and/or risk factors influencing prevalence change?)
  » What are the strengths/limitations of these approaches?
  » What else could be done to understand ASD trends using this dataset?
  » What else is needed to understand ASD trends?

10:50–11:05 ....Break

11:05–12:30 ....Lessons from other conditions and analytic methodologies

- Cancer — R. Etzioni
- Parkinson's — C. Tanner
- Asthma — M. King
- Schizophrenia — E. Susser
- Simulation Studies — S. Galea

Given a change in prevalence/ incidence, what has been done to understand the reason(s)?

- Brief overview of evidence of prevalence changes.
- What factors contribute to the change in prevalence over time? (is it possible to distinguish the relative contribution of various intrinsic identification, extrinsic identification, and/or risk factors influencing prevalence change?)
- What are the strengths/ limitations of these approaches?
- What lessons may be important when looking at reasons for ASD trends?

12:30–1:00 ....Open Comment

1:00–1:20 ....Pick up lunch and transition to Panel Breakouts

1:20–2:45 ....Panel Discussion Breakouts

Panel 1 – Utility of ASD Prevalence Information (Room 117)

Panel Chair: *A. Singer*
Recorder: *C. Arneson*
Panelists: *C. Cunniff, W. Zahorodny, R. Kirby, M. Lopez, R. Grinker, D. Mandell*, L. Grossman*, W. Dunaway, M. Rosanoff, J. Zimmerman, B. Mulvihill, J Charles*

- What does having ASD prevalence information do for stakeholders (parents, professionals, people with

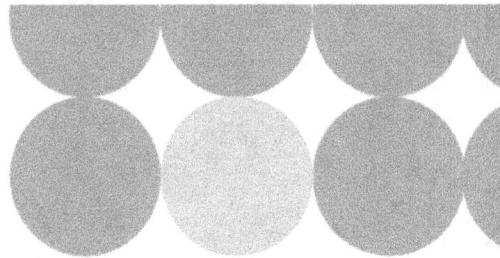

ASD, policy makers, service providers)?

- How are stakeholders actually using ASD prevalence information?
- What types of ASD prevalence information and descriptions of the population are useful to stakeholders?
- What questions do stakeholders expect epidemiology and prevalence reports, in particular, to answer?

Panel 2 – Other US-Based ASD Data (Room 255)

Panel Chair: *L. Croen*
Recorder: *L. King*
Panelists: *P. Shattuck, P. Bearman, M. Kogan, S. Visser, I. Hertz-Piciotto, L. Miller, A. Bakian, K. Van Naarden Braun, L. Lee, T. Baroud, P. Bell, R. Etzioni, Y. Kim*

- What are the top 3 immediate (1–2 year) priority analyses needed to understand ASD trends using existing US-based datasets?
- What are the top 3 next (3–5 year) priority analyses needed to understand ASD trends using existing US-based datasets?
- Can these data systems be enhanced (analyses, data collection, others) to better answer questions about changing prevalence of ASDs? If yes, how? If no, why not and what else is needed?

Panel 3 – ADDM Network Data (Room 257)

Panel Chair: *G. Dawson*
Recorder: *K. Phillips*
Panelists: *S. Galea, G. McGwin, O. Devine, A. Correa, M. Zack, P. Yoon, M. Maenner, J. Daniels, L. Schieve, S. Pettygrove, M. Wingate, J. E. Robison, P. C. Marvin*

- What are the top 3 immediate (1 -2 year) priority analyses needed to understand ASD trends using existing ADDM data?
- What are the top 3 next (3-5 year) priority analyses needed to understand ASD trends using existing ADDM data?
- Can the ADDM Network be enhanced (analyses, data collection, others) to better answer questions about changing prevalence of ASDs? If yes, how? If no, why not and what else is needed?

Panel 4 –What else could be done to understand ASD Trends? (Room B1/B2)

Panel Chair: *M. Durkin*
Recorder: *R. Fitzgerald*
Panelists: *K. Crider, E. Susser, C. Lawler, C. Tanner, M. King, S. Shapira, D. Schendel, J. Nicholas, W. McMahon, J. Constantino, C. Newschaffer, L. Perner, M. Blaxill, E. London, G. Windham, K. Merikangas*

- Can the question of the relative contribution of identification and/or risk factors on ASD prevalence in the last 20 years be answered?
  - » If not, why?
  - » If yes, what are the 3 primary questions which need to be addressed by epidemiology?
- How can the ASD field work with other fields / conditions to evaluate trends (comparison to other conditions, sharing methodology, analytic techniques, etc.)? How best can that be accomplished (give specific

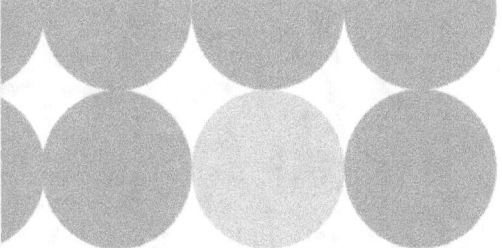

conditions with possible analyses/activities)?

- What else is needed for the ASD larger field to understand reasons for trends?

2:45–3:00 .... Break

3:00–5:00 .... Report from Each Panel (Aud A)
Facilitator: P. Yoon

- 3:00–4:45 .... For Panel 1, 2, 3, and 4
  - » 10 minute summary report for each panel
  - » 15 minute Larger Panel Discussion
- 4:45–5:00 .... Meeting adjournment

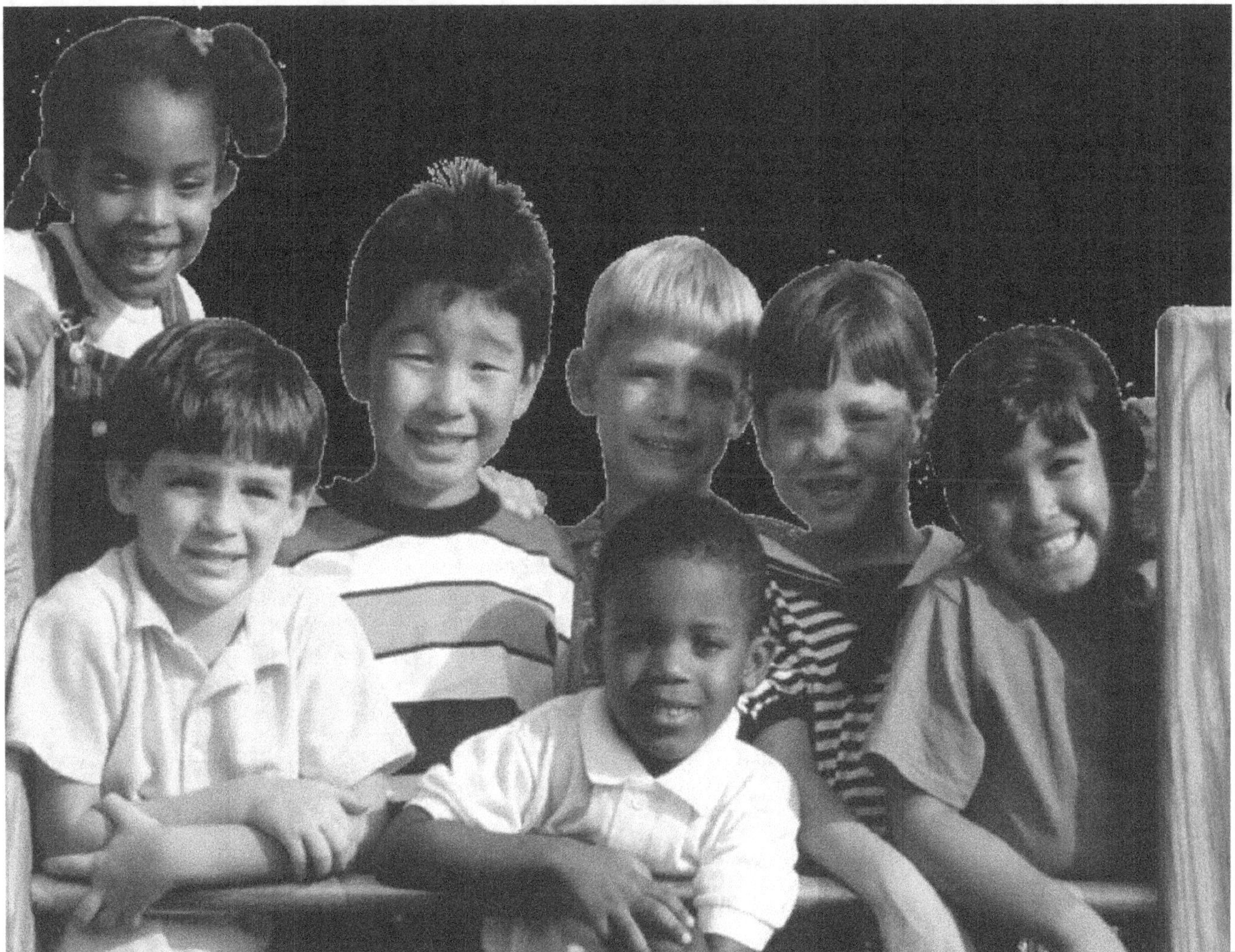

Appendix B:
Panelist Biographies

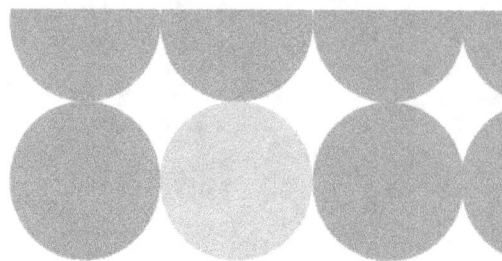

Amanda V. Bakian, MS, PhD, is the epidemiologist and data manager for the Utah Registry of Autism and Developmental Disabilities (URADD) and the Utah ADDM Network site. She has collaborated on a variety of research studies investigating the prenatal, perinatal, neonatal, socio-demographic, and environmental risk factors associated with ASDs and intellectual disabilities.

Thaer Baroud, BSN, MA, MHSA, is a senior epidemiologist with the Arkansas comprehensive tobacco control program and he is the epidemiologist for the Arkansas ADDM Network site. He has worked as an epidemiologist at the Arkansas Center for Health Statistics.

Peter Bearman, PhD, is the Director of the Lazarsfeld Center for the Social Sciences, the Cole Professor of Social Science, and Co-Director of the Health & Society Scholars Program at Columbia University. He is currently investigating the social determinants of the autism epidemic. He has researched topics including adolescent sexual networks, networks of disease transmission, genetic influences on same-sex preference, and historical sociology.

Peter Bell, MBA, is Executive Vice President for Programs and Services at Autism Speaks and the father of a son with autism. He oversees the foundation's government relations and family services activities and also serves as an advisor to the science division. Mr. Bell was president and CEO of Cure Autism Now following a marketing career at McNeil Consumer & Specialty Pharmaceuticals, a member of the Johnson & Johnson family of companies.

Mark Blaxill, MBA, is the father of a daughter with autism, editor-at-large for Age of Autism, a director of SafeMinds, and a frequent speaker at autism conferences. He writes often on autism, science, and public policy. In his professional career, he is managing partner for 3LP Advisors, an advisory firm focused on intellectual property transactions.

Coleen A. Boyle, PhD, MSHyg, is the Director of the National Center on Birth Defects and Developmental Disabilities (NCBDDD) at CDC. She has worked on public health issues such as agent orange and cancer. Her interest and expertise is in the epidemiology and prevention of birth defects and developmental disabilities.

Jane Charles, MD, is a Developmental-Behavioral Pediatrician in the Department of Pediatrics at Medical University of South Carolina. Her areas of specialization are in the fields of ASDs and intellectual disabilities. For the past ten years, she has been Co-Principal Investigator for the South Carolina ADDM Network site.

Prisca Chen Marvin, JD, is the mother of a daughter with autism, a member of the Visiting Committee at Massachusetts Institute of Technology's Brain and Cognitive Science Department, a board member of REACH at the University of Iowa, and a Member of the Executive Council of the Associates of the Yale Child Study Center.

John N. Constantino, MD, is the Blanche F. Ittleson Professor of Psychiatry and Pediatrics at Washington University, Associate Director of a Eunice Kennedy Shriver Intellectual and Developmental Disabilities Research Center at the Washington University School of Medicine, and Director of the School's Division of Child Psychiatry. In addition to his role as Principal Investigator of the Missouri ADDM Network site, he leads a federally-funded program in autism research that is centered on a prospective longitudinal study of sibling pairs in families affected by autism.

Adolfo Correa, MD, MPH, PhD, is a Medical Officer and Birth Defects Surveillance Team Lead with the CDC's National Center on Birth Defects and Developmental Disabilities, Birth Defects Branch. He has worked extensively with the Metropolitan Atlanta Congenital Defects Program (MACDP). His current work focuses on surveillance of congenital heart defects and on the epidemiology of maternal diabetes and birth defects.

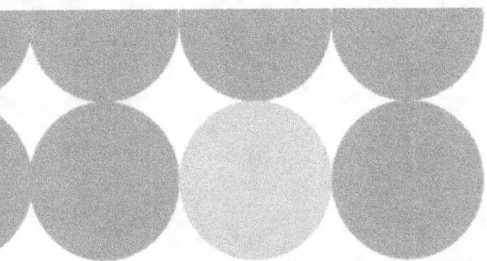

Krista S. Crider, MA, PhD, is a Geneticist with the CDC's National Center on Birth Defects and Developmental Disabilities, Pediatric Genetics Team. She has worked on epigenetics changes in DNA methylation and folic acid supplementation, antibiotic use and the risk of birth defects, trends in trisomies, and genetics of preterm birth among other projects with the National Birth Defects Prevention Study, Metropolitan Congenital Defects Program, and the China collaboration.

Lisa A. Croen, PhD, is a Senior Research Scientist and the Director of the Kaiser Permanente® Autism Research Program. Currently, she is leading or collaborating on several federally funded autism studies, including the Study to Explore Early Development (SEED), the Early Autism Risk Longitudinal Investigation Study (EARLI), the Early Markers for Autism Study (EMA), the California Autism Twins Study (CATS), and the Mental Health Research Network Autism Registry project.

Christopher Cunniff, MD, FACMG, FAAP, is a Professor of Pediatrics and Chief of the Section of Medical and Molecular Genetics at the University of Arizona, College of Medicine. His research focuses on public health genetics and the surveillance of developmental disabilities including ASDs, intellectual disability, muscular dystrophy, and fetal alcohol syndrome.

Julie Daniels, PhD, is a pediatric epidemiologist and Associate Professor in the Department of Epidemiology and Maternal and Child Health at University of North Carolina at Chapel Hill. She is the Principal Investigator of the North Carolina ADDM Network site and the CDC's Study to Explore Early Development (SEED) North Carolina site since 2002. Her research focuses on perinatal exposures, specifically nutrition and environmental exposures that may be associated with child health and development.

Geraldine Dawson, PhD, is Chief Science Officer for Autism Speaks, Research Professor of Psychiatry at the University of North Carolina at Chapel Hill, Adjunct Professor of Psychiatry at Columbia University, and Professor Emeritus of Psychology at University of Washington. She is a licensed clinical psychologist who has published extensively on autism, focusing on early detection and intervention and early patterns of brain dysfunction.

Owen Devine, PhD, is a Mathematical Statistician with the CDC's National Center on Birth Defects and Developmental Disabilities. He provides guidance on the analysis of epidemiologic data related to birth defects and developmental disabilities. His areas of interest included Bayesian methods, missing and miss measured data, and the interface of mathematical modeling and statistical techniques as applied to public health.

Wolf F. Dunaway works for the federal government as an Information Technology Specialist. He speaks at various colleges, universities, and symposiums on issues associated with autism and other disabilities and helps others better understand childhood autism through his own autism life experiences.

Maureen Durkin, PhD, DrPH, is a Professor of Population Health Sciences and Pediatrics and Waisman Center Investigator at the University of Wisconsin-Madison and the Principal Investigator of the Wisconsin ADDM Network site. She is an epidemiologist specializing in population-based studies of the frequency, prevention, antecedents, and consequences of developmental disabilities.

Ruth Etzioni, PhD, is a biostatistician and a full member at the Fred Hutchinson Cancer Research Center in Seattle. She studies population trends in prostate cancer incidence and mortality and is one of the principal investigators on the National Cancer Institute's Cancer Intervention and Surveillance Modeling Network. She is currently adapting models for use in policy development for PSA screening.

Sandro Galea, MD, MPH, DrPH, is a physician, epidemiologist, and the Anna Cheskis Gelman and Murray Charles Gelman Professor and Chair of the Department of Epidemiology at Columbia University's Mailman School of Public Health. He has conducted large population-based studies in several countries,

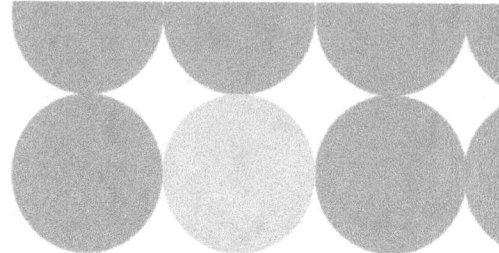

and his primary research has been on the causes of mental disorders, substance abuse and on the role of traumatic events in shaping population health.

Roy Richard Grinker, PhD, is Professor of Anthropology at the George Washington University and editor-in-chief of The Anthropological Quarterly. He has published on topics such as the ethnic conflict in central Africa, intellectual history of African Studies, north-south Korean relations, and autism. He was a collaborator on a prevalence study of autism in South Korea and is a Co-Investigator on an NIMH-funded project entitled "Early Social Communication Characteristics of ASD in Diverse Cultures in the US and Africa".

Lee Grossman*, CAE, was the President and CEO of the Autism Society of America through early 2011 and the father of a son with autism. He has more than 20 years of experience with autism related issues, notably autism services and supports, adult issues, education, and research. He has served on numerous government and non-government advisory boards related to autism. Mr. Grossman has owned and operated a small business specializing in marketing, distribution, and consulting for medical manufacturers throughout the Pacific Basin.

Irva Hertz-Picciotto, PhD, is a Professor of Health Sciences at the University of California, Davis. She has published extensively on the effects of environmental exposures on pregnancy and child development. She is the Principal Investigator of CHARGE (Childhood Autism Risks from Genetics and Environment) Study, the first large, comprehensive population-based study of environmental factors in autism, and MARBLES (Markers of Autism Risk in Babies – Learning Early Signs), to search for early biologic markers that will predict autism.

Young Shin Kim, MD, MPH, PhD, is a researcher at Yale University. Her major research efforts focus on school bullying, the epidemiology of childhood onset neuropsychiatric disorders, and the genetic epidemiology of childhood onset neuropsychiatric disorders. She was the lead author on an epidemiological study of ASD prevalence in South Korea.

Michael King MSW, PhD, is a Commander in the US Public Health Service and an epidemiologist with the CDC's National Center for Environmental Health, Division of Environmental Hazards & Health Effects, Air Pollution and Respiratory Health Branch. His research has focused on using national surveys to monitor asthma-related morbidity, health-service use, and other respiratory health outcomes, including unintentional carbon monoxide poisoning.

Russell S. Kirby, PhD, MS, FACE, is Professor and Marrell-endowed Chair in the Department of Community and Family Health, College of Public Health, University of South Florida. He is a pediatric and perinatal epidemiologist with extensive experience in population health informatics and public health surveillance of birth defects and developmental disabilities and has been involved with the ADDM Network since 2002.

Michael D. Kogan, PhD, is Director of the Office of Epidemiology, Policy, and Evaluation for the US Health Resources and Services Administration's Maternal and Child Health Bureau. He also directs the US National Surveys of Children's Health and the National Surveys of Children with Special Health Care Needs. He has published over 100 articles and book chapters on numerous topics in pediatric and perinatal epidemiology, including the prevalence of ASDs, as well as the health care experiences of families with children who have an ASD.

Cindy Lawler, PhD, is a Program Director in the Division of Extramural Research and Training at the National Institute for Environmental Health Sciences (NIEHS), one of the National Institutes of Health. She is the NIEHS representative for extramural autism activities; this includes responsibilities as a program official for the NIH-funded Early Autism Risk Longitudinal Investigation (EARLI) study.

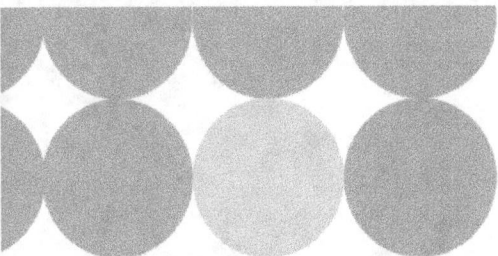

Li-Ching Lee, PhD, ScM, is a Research Scientist with the Department of Epidemiology at the Johns Hopkins Bloomberg School of Public Health at the Johns Hopkins University. She has a background is in psychiatric epidemiology and a research interest in developmental disabilities in the US, China, and Taiwan. She has been involved with Maryland ADDM Network site since early in its inception and is currently the Principal Investigator.

Eric London, MD, is trained as a general psychiatrist and has a son with autism. He and his wife started the National Alliance for Autism Research (NAAR) in 1994, which later merged with Autism Speaks. He now serves on the Board of the Autism Science Foundation. Dr. London was the Director of the Autism Treatment Laboratory at the New York State Institute for Basic Research, and is now the Research Director at the the Center for Discovery in Harris, New York. His primary interests are in very early identification of autism and creating novel methods for autism treatment research.

Maya Lopez, MD, is a Developmental-Behavioral Pediatrician and Assistant Professor in the Developmental-Behavioral and Rehabilitative Pediatrics in the Department of Pediatrics College of Medicine at University of Arkansas Medical Sciences. She is the current Principal Investigator on the Autism Treatment Network (ATN) Grant for her institution and is Co-Principal Investigator for the Arkansas ADDM Network site.

David S. Mandell*, ScD, is Associate Professor of Psychiatry and Pediatrics at the University of Pennsylvania School of Medicine, an Associate Director of the Center for Mental Health Policy and Services Research, and Associate Director of the Center for Autism Research at The Children's Hospital of Philadelphia. The goal of his research is to improve the quality of care individuals with autism receive in their communities.

Matthew Maenner is a PhD candidate at the University of Wisconsin and works as an epidemiologist and data manager for the Wisconsin site of the ADDM network. He is currently funded by the Autism Science Foundation to explore the phenotypic heterogeneity of autism and its relationship to early identification.

Gerald McGwin, PhD, is a Professor and Vice Chairman in the Department of Epidemiology in the School of Public Health at the University of Alabama at Birmingham. He is an associate editor for the American Journal of Epidemiology, and has a lengthy and distinguished scientific reputation as a researcher, having authored or co-authored over 300 peer-reviewed manuscripts, with an emphasis on injury and ophthalmic epidemiology.

William M. McMahon, MD, is the Chairman of the Department of Psychiatry and a Professor of Psychiatry, Pediatrics, Psychology and Educational Psychology at the University of Utah. His research interests include the genetics and epidemiology of autism, Tourette's Disorder, nicotine addiction, and suicide. He is a Senior Investigator for the Autism Genome Project and is currently Principal Investigator of an Autism Speaks funded follow-up study of the Utah Autism Studies sample.

Kathleen Ries Merikangas, PhD, is a Senior Investigator and Chief of the Genetic Epidemiology Branch in the Intramural Research Program at the National Institute of Mental Health (NIMH). Her research interests have included clinical research on affective disorders and genetic epidemiology.

Lisa Miller, MD, MSPH, is the director of the Disease Control and Environmental Epidemiology Division at the Colorado Department of Public Health and Environment. She is the Co-Principal Investigator of the CDC-funded Colorado sites of the ADDM Network site and the Study to Explore Early Development (SEED). She currently directs epidemiologic programs concerning communicable diseases, environmental health, autism, and muscular dystrophy.

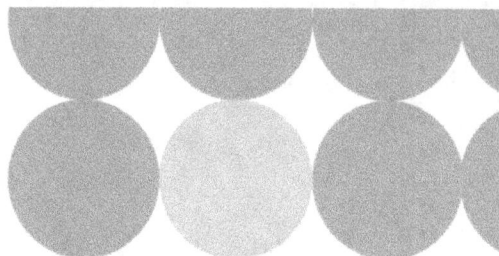

Beverly Mulvihill MEd, PhD, is currently an Associate Professor in the Department of Health Care Organization and Policy and a Research Scientist with the Civitan International Research Center at the University of Alabama at Birmingham. She has been Principal Investigator or Co-Principal Investigator of the Alabama ADDM Network site since 2008. Her research interests include child development; children with and at-risk for disabilities, especially autism spectrum disorders; and early identification, intervention, and inclusion for children in need of special services.

Craig Newschaffer, PhD, is Professor and Chairman of the Department of Epidemiology and Biostatistics at Drexel University School of Public Health. He leads an NIH-funded EARLI Study, which is designed specifically to study pre, peri- and neonatal autism risk factors and biomarkers. He is also a Principal Investigator on other major autism epidemiology initiatives. Prior to focusing his research on autism, he worked extensively in cancer epidemiology.

Joyce S. Nicholas PhD, is an Associate Professor in the Medical University of South Carolina's Department of Medicine, Division of Biostatistics and Epidemiology, with a dual appointment in the Department of Neurosciences. She specializes in neuro-epidemiology, in particular neurodevelopmental and other neurologic conditions. She is a Co-Principal Investigator for the South Carolina ADDM Network site.

Lars Perner, PhD, is an Assistant Professor of Clinical Marketing at the Marshall School of Business of the University of Southern California. His research interests focus on consumer behavior, "win-win" deals, non-profit marketing, and autism subtypes. He currently serves as Chair of the Panel of Persons on the Spectrum of Autism Advisors for the Autism Society.

Sydney Pettygrove, PhD, is an Assistant Professor of Epidemiology, College of Public Health, at the University of Arizona, Tucson. She primarily works on the effects of environmental and occupational exposures on reproductive outcomes including birth defects and developmental disabilities. She is the Co-Principal Investigator of the Arizona ADDM Network site.

Catherine E. Rice, PhD, is an Epidemiologist with CDC's National Center on Birth Defects and Developmental Disabilities, Developmental Disabilities Branch and has worked with people with an ASD through teaching, diagnostic assessment, intervention, training, and research. She has been a lead scientist with the ADDM Network since 2001. She works on public health programs related to autism with specific interests in early identification, diagnosis, prevalence, and risk factors for autism.

John Elder Robison is a self-identified "free range" Aspergian male. He is the founder of a specialty automobile company, pioneered specialty guitars for the band KISS, and worked on some of the first talking toys for Milton Bradley. He serves as adjunct faculty in the department of Communication Sciences and Disorders at Elms College in Massachusetts and has served on several national autism science boards as a community member. He is the author of Look Me in the Eye: My life with Asperger's.

Michael Rosanoff, MPH, is the Associate Director of Public Health Research and Scientific Review for Autism Speaks. He is a member of Autism Speaks etiology team and manages the organization's epidemiology and public health research grants. He is also the staff lead in overseeing the International Autism Epidemiology Network (IAEN) and is part of the development team for the Global Autism Public Health Initiative (GAPH).

Diana E. Schendel, PhD, is Lead Health Scientist and Epidemiology Team Lead with the CDC's National Center for Birth Defects and Developmental Disabilities, Developmental Disabilities Branch. She serves as Principal Investigator for the Centers for Autism and Developmental Disabilities Research and Epidemiology (CADDRE) which includes the Study to Explore Early Development (SEED). She is Project Lead for the International Collaboration for Autism Registry Epidemiology (iCARE). Her research interests include risk factors for cerebral palsy and autism.

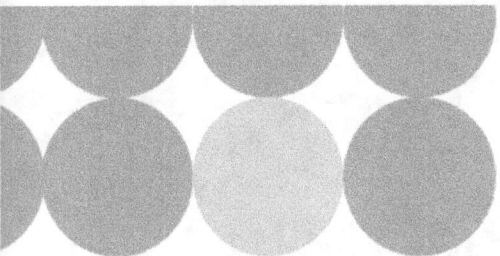

Laura A. Schieve, PhD is an Epidemiologist with the CDC's National Center on Birth Defects and Developmental Disabilities, Developmental Disabilities Branch. Dr. Schieve is one of the Principal Investigators on the CDC's Study to Explore Early Development (SEED). Her current research includes prevalence of autism and other developmental disabilities, maternal and perinatal risk factors for developmental disability, health care needs and family functioning in families with a disabled child, and epidemiologic methods for assessing maternal and child risk factors in populations.

Stuart K. Shapira, MD, PhD, is a Medical Officer with CDC's National Center on Birth Defects and Developmental Disabilities, Pediatric Genetics Team. He is an investigator on the CDC Study to Explore Early Development (SEED). His current interests include birth defects epidemiologic research, dysmorphology of autism, gene and nutritional interactions for adverse reproductive outcomes, and newborn screening.

Paul T. Shattuck, PhD, is an Assistant Professor at the George Warren Brown School of Social Work at Washington University in St. Louis. Dr. Shattuck conducts research aimed at improving systems of care and services for people with autism and their families. He is especially interested in two key service transitions: getting a diagnosis in early childhood and exiting high school in adolescence.

Ezra Susser, MD, DrPH, is Professor of Epidemiology and Psychiatry at Columbia University. Dr. Susser heads the Imprints Center for Genetic and Environmental Lifecourse Studies, a collaborative birth cohort research program in which epidemiologists seek to uncover the causes of a broad range of disease and health outcomes, including psychiatric and neurodevelopmental disorders, obesity, cardiovascular disease, reproductive performance, and breast and ovarian cancers. His own studies focus on schizophrenia and autism.

Alison Singer, MBA, is Co-Founder and President of the Autism Science Foundation, a not-for-profit organization that funds autism research and serves to increase awareness of ASDs and the needs of individuals and families affected by autism. She has been very involved in advocacy for autism as the mother of a child with autism and legal guardian of her adult brother with autism. She spent 14 years at CNBC and NBC in a variety of positions, including vice president of programming in NBC's cable and business development division and as a producer. Ms. Singer has served on several research, advocacy, and government advisory boards for autism.

Caroline M. Tanner, MD, PhD, FAAN, is Director of Clinical Research at the Parkinson's Institute in Sunnyvale, California, a Visiting Professor at Xuan Wu Hospital and Capital University in Beijing, China, and an Adjunct Professor in the Department of Health Research and Policy at Stanford University. Her current research includes epidemiologic investigations of the genetic and environmental determinants of Parkinson's disease, multiple system atrophy, dystonia, Huntington's disease and essential tremor in a variety of populations in the US.

Kim Van Naarden Braun, PhD, is an Epidemiologist with the CDC's National Center on Birth Defects and Developmental Disabilities, Developmental Disabilities Branch and with the New Jersey Department of Health and Senior Services. She is the Principal Investigator for the Metropolitan Atlanta Developmental Disabilities Surveillance Program (MADDSP) and also serves an epidemiologist for the ADDM Network and the ADDM Cerebral Palsy Network. Research interests include developmental disabilities, perinatal epidemiology, genetic epidemiology, environmental health, and child health and development.

Susanna Visser, MS, is the lead Epidemiologist with the CDC's National Center on Birth Defects and Developmental Disabilities, Child Development Studies Team. Her current research interests include population-based epidemiological studies of neurobehavioral and mental health conditions, including ADHD and Tourette Syndrome, medication treatment among youth with ADHD, and factors associated with ADHD medication treatment.

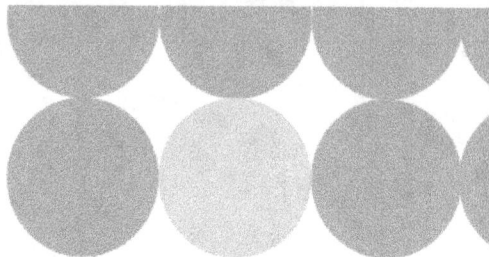

Gayle Windham, PhD, is a Research Scientist and Chief of the Epidemiological Surveillance Section at the California Department of Public Health in the Division of Environmental and Occupational Disease Control. She currently works with the Centers for Autism and Developmental Disabilities Research (CADDRE) team and is the lead investigator on a study of early ASD prevalence in California. Her areas of research and expertise include children's health in relation to environmental risk factors, pregnancy outcomes such as spontaneous abortion and fetal growth, and other aspects of reproductive health including puberty, infertility, and menstrual function.

Martha S. Wingate, DrPH, is an Assistant Professor at University of Alabama at Birmingham in the Department of Health Care Organization and Policy. She is the Co-Principal Investigator of the Alabama ADDM Network site. Much of her work focuses on preterm birth, fetal and infant mortality, racial and ethnic disparities in birth outcomes, and health policies related to pregnancy and infant health.

Marshalyn Yeargin-Allsopp, MD, is a Medical Epidemiologist and Branch Chief with the CDC's National Center on Birth Defects and Developmental Disabilities, Developmental Disabilities Branch. She designed and implemented the first U.S. population-based study of developmental disabilities in school-age children in an urban area, which has served as the basis for the ADDM Network and the Centers for Autism and Developmental Disabilities Research and Epidemiology (CADDRE). She has presented internationally and published extensively on the epidemiology of developmental disabilities, including autism and cerebral palsy.

Paula Yoon, MPH, ScD, is currently the Team Lead for the Health Services Research and Registries Team in the Division for Heart Disease and Stroke Prevention, Epidemiology and Surveillance Branch. She is also leading an initiative to establish a National Cardiovascular Disease Surveillance System. She is the Chair of the Surveillance Science Advisory Group at CDC and is spearheading an effort to develop an agency-wide surveillance report to track the impact of health care reform on prevention in health care.

Matthew Zack, MD, is a Medical Epidemiologist with the CDC's National Center for Chronic Disease Prevention and Health Promotion, Division of Adult and Community Health, State Support, Arthritis, Epilepsy, & Quality of Life Branch. He has worked extensively on issues related to chronic diseases and environmental health.

Walter Zahorodny, PhD, is a clinical psychologist and Assistant Professor of Pediatrics at the New Jersey Medical School. He has over twenty years of experience in pediatric neurodevelopment and is the Principal Investigator of the New Jersey ADDM Network site for population-based ASD surveillance system. He is a founding member of the New Jersey Medical School Autism Center and was instrumental in development of the New Jersey Governor's Council on Medical Research and Treatment of Autism.

Judith Pinborough Zimmerman, PhD, CCC, is an Assistant Professor in the Department of Psychiatry at the University of Utah. She is the for the Utah Registry for Autism and Developmental Disabilities (URADD) and the Principal Investigator for the Utah ADDM Network site. She is particularly interested in the utility of ASD prevalence data for state Maternal and Child Health Programs.

RECORDERS

Carrie Arneson, MSc, serves as Project Coordinator for the Wisconsin ADDM Network site located at the Waisman Center at University of Wisconsin-Madison.

Jon Baio, EdS, is an Epidemiologist with the CDC's National Center on Birth Defects and Developmental Disabilities, Developmental Disabilities Branch. He currently serves as Principal Investigator on the ADDM Network, studying the prevalence of autism and other developmental disabilities in several communities throughout the U.S.

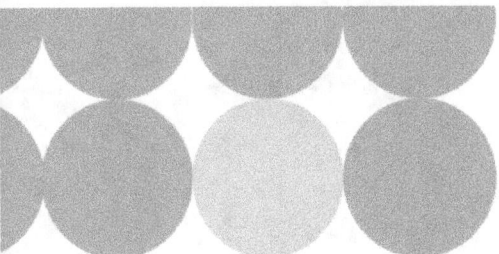

Thomas A. Bartenfeld, PhD, specializes in program evaluation with the CDC's National Center on Birth Defects and Developmental Disabilities. His most recent work has focused on using evaluation to promote information to action and organizational integration with NCBDDD's surveillance, research, and prevention programs.

Robert Fitzgerald, MPH is currently a staff scientist in the Department of Psychiatry at the Washington University School of Medicine in St. Louis, and is a PhD candidate in Epidemiology at the St. Louis University School of Public Health. He has served as Project Coordinator for the Missouri ADDM Network site since its inception in 2003 and has served as Co-Principal Investigator since April of 2009.

Lydia King, PhD, is an Assistant Professor of Pediatrics at the Medical University of South Carolina and is an Epidemiologist specializing in ASDs. She has served as the Project Coordinator for the South Carolina ADDM site since 2003. She is also Faculty Director for the Global Education Masters in Clinical Research Program.

Keydra Phillips, MSc, is a Health Scientist with the CDC's National Center on Birth Defects and Developmental Disabilities, Developmental Disabilities Branch. She is a member of an interdisciplinary team of researchers of the ADDM Network, and her research interests include public health informatics and surveillance of chronic diseases.

Andria M. Ratchford, MSPH, has served as the Project Coordinator for the Colorado ADDM Network site at the Colorado Department of Public Health and Environment since 2002. She has considerable surveillance and project management experience through her experience with ADDM and the Colorado Center of Autism and Developmental Disabilities Research and Epidemiology (CADDRE) activities.

Anita Washington, MPH, is a Research Public Health Analyst with Research Triangle Institute (RTI) as part of the Atlanta Regional Office. For the past 6 years, she has been working as a contract employee in the role of the ADDM Network Project Coordinator for CDC's National Center on Birth Defects and Developmental Disabilities, Division of Birth Defects and Developmental Disabilities, Developmental Disabilities Branch.

Invited participant unable to attend remotely or in-person at last minute due to unforeseen circumstances.

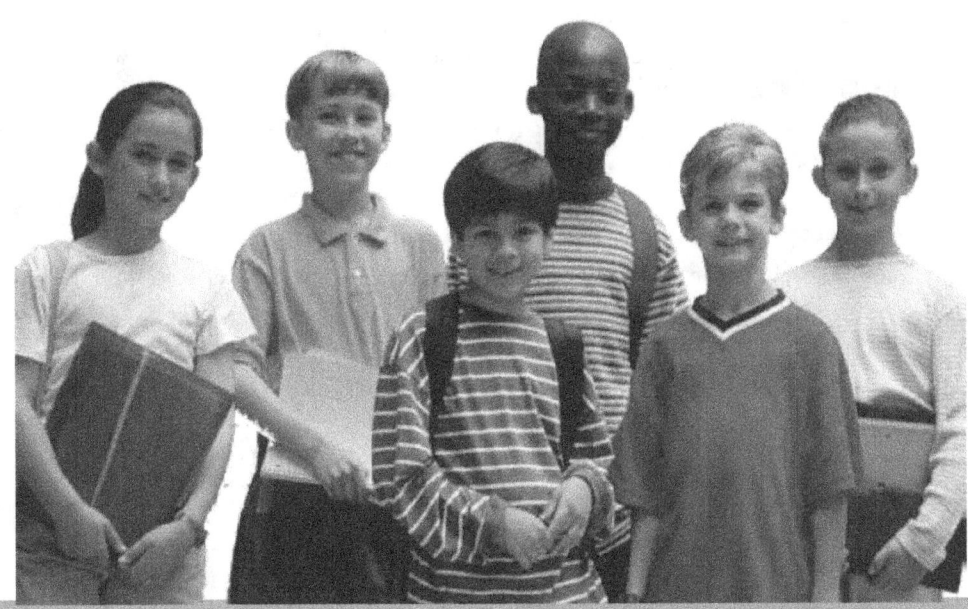

Appendix C: Reference List

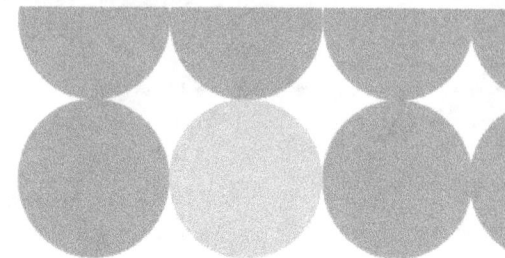

References were compiled based on panel member nominations for suggested background reading on ASD prevalence.

Panel members were asked to read the articles indicated with an * prior to the workshop.

ASD Prevalence Reviews

* Blaxill, M. (2004). What's going on? the question of time trends in autism. *Public Health Reports,* 119(6), 536-551.

* Fombonne, E. (2009). Epidemiology of pervasive developmental disorders. *Pediatric Research,* 65(6), 591-598.

Gernsbacher, M., Dawson, M., Goldsmith, H. (2005). Three reasons not to believe in an autism epidemic. *Current Directions in Psychological Science,* 14(2), 55-58.

* Leonard, H., Dixon, G., Whitehouse, A., Bourke, J., Aiberti, K., Nassar, N., et. al. (2010). Unpacking the complex nature of the autism epidemic. *Research in Autism Spectrum Disorders,* 4(4), 548-554.

* McDonald, M., Paul, J. (2010). Timing of increased autistic disorder cumulative incidence. *Environmental Science & Technology,* 44(6), 2112-2118.

Rutter, M. (2005). Incidence of autism spectrum disorders: changes over time and their meaning. *Acta Paediatrica,* 94(1), 2-15.

* Russell, G., Kelly, S., Golding, J. (2010). A qualitative analysis of lay beliefs about the aetiology and prevalence of autistic spectrum disorders. *Child: care, health and development,* 36(3), 431-436. (*of note for Panel 1*)

Society for Research in Child Development (SRCD). (2010). Social policy report on the autism spectrum disorders. SRCD SocialPolicy Report, 24(2). (of note for Panel 1)

Wazana, A., Breshnahan, M., Kline, J. (2007). The autism epidemic: fact or artifact?. *Journal of the American Academy of Child and Adolescent Psychiatry,* 46(6), 721-730.

ASDs Background

Abrahams, B., Geschwind, D. (2008). Advances in autism genetics: on the threshold of a new neurobiology. Nat Rev Genet., 9(5),341-55.

American Academy of Pediatrics Council on Children with Disabilities. (2006). Identifying infants and young children with developmental disorders in the medical home: an algorithm for developmental surveillance and screening. *Pediatrics,* 118:405–20.

* Constantino, J., Todd, R. (2003). Autistic traits in the general population: a twin study. *Archives of General Psychiatry,* 60, 524–530.

Constantino, J., Zhang, Y., Frazier, T., Abbacchi, A., Law, P. (2010). Sibling recurrence and the genetic epidemiology of autism. *American Journal of Psychiatry,* 167, 1349–1356.

Daniels JL. (2006). Autism and the environment. Environmental Health Perspectives, Jul;114(7):A396.

* Grinker, R. (2010). In retrospect: the five lives of the psychiatry manual. *Nature,* 468, 168-170.

Happé, F., Ronald, A. (2008). The 'fractionable autism triad': a review of evidence from behavioural, genetic, cognitive and neural research. *Neuropsychology Review,* 18(4), 287–304.

* Herbert, M. (2010). Contributions of the environment and environmentally vulnerable physiology to autism spectrum disorders. *Current Opinion in Neurology,* 23, 103–110.

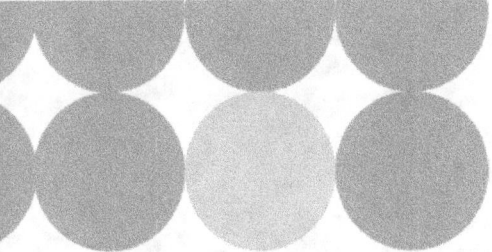

Landrigan PJ. What causes autism? Exploring the environmental contribution. Current Opinion Pediatrics. 2010 Apr;22(2):219-25.

* Lichtenstein, P., Carlström, E., Råstam, M., Gillberg, C., Anckarsäter, H. (2010). The genetics of autism spectrum disorders and related neuropsychiatric disorders in childhood. *The American Journal of Psychiatry,* 167(11), 1357-1363.

Rondeau, E., Klein, L., Masse, A., Bodeau, N., Cohen, D., Guilé, J. (2011). Is pervasive developmental disorder not otherwise specified less stable than autistic disorder? a meta-analysis. Journal of Autism and Developmental Disorders,41(9), 1267-1276.

U.S. Department of Education Autism Trends (of note for Panel 2)

Becker, K. (2010). Letters – autism and urbanization. *American Journal of Public Health,* 100(7), 1156-1159.

Harrington, J. (2010). The actual prevalence of autism: are we there yet?. *Pediatrics,* 126(5), e1257-1258.

* Individuals with Disabilities Education Act (IDEA) Definitions for Special Education Eligibility.

Individuals with Disabilities Education Act (IDEA) Data. Washington, DC: U.S. Department of Education , Office of Special Education Programs; 2009. Number of children served under IDEA by disability and age group through 2007. https://www.ideadata.org/PartBData.asp.

MacFarlane, J., Kanaya, T. (2009). What does it mean to be autistic? inter-state variation in special education criteria for autism services. *Journal of Child and Family Studies,* 18, 662-669

* Maenner, M., Durkin, M. (2010). Trends in the prevalence of autism on the basis of special education data. *Pediatric,* 126(5), 1018-1025.

* Newschaffer, C., Falb, M., Gurney, J. (2005). National autism prevalence trends from united states special education data. *Pediatrics,* 115(3), 277-282.

* Shattuck, P. (2006). The contribution of diagnostic substitution to the growing administrative prevalence of autism in us special education. *Pediatrics,* 117(4), 1028-1037.

California Developmental Disabilities Services (CA DDS) (of note for Panel 2)

* CA DDS Summary Documents

   Bakian A. Summary of CA DDS Autism Data.
   CA DDS CEDR Form.

Cavagnaro, A. (2009). Autistic spectrum disorders changes in the california caseload an update: june 1987-june 2007. *California Department of Developmental Services,* 19(6), 536-551.

* Hertz-Picciotto, I., Delwiche, L. (2009). The rise in autism and the role of age at diagnosis. *Epidemiology,* 20, 84–90.

* King, M., Bearman, P. (2009). Diagnostic change and the increased prevalence of autism. *International Journal of Epidemiology,* 38(5), 1224-1234. (commentaries by Charman, Formbonne, Hertz-Picciotto, Rutter, and response).

* Liu, K., Zerubavel, N., Bearman, P. (2010). Social demographic change and autism. *Demography,* 47(2), 327-343.

Liu, K., King, M., Bearman, P. (2010). Social influence and the autism epidemic. *American Journal of Sociology,* 115(5), 1387-1434.

Schechter, R., Grether, J. (2008). Continuing increases in autism reported to california's developmental

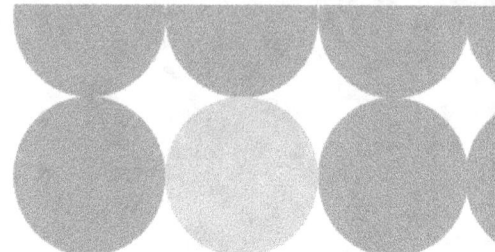

services system: mercury in retrograde. *Archives of General Psychiatry,* 65(1), 19-24.

* Shelton, J., Tancredi, D., Hertz-Picciotto I. (2010). Independent and dependent contributions of advanced maternal and paternal ages to autism risk. *Autism Research,* 3(1), 30-39.

* Van Meter, K., Christiansen, L., Delwiche, L., Azari, R., Carpenter, T., Hertz-Picciotto, I. (2010). Geographic distribution of autism in california: A retrospective birth cohort analysis. *Autism Research,* 3(1), 19-29.

Autism and Developmental Disabilities Monitoring (ADDM) Network (of note for Panel 3)
ADDM Network Summary Documents

Evaluating Change Summary Grid
ADDM Network Community Report (2009). (of note for Panel 1)

* Centers for Disease Control and Prevention . (2009). Prevalence of autism spectrum disorders - autism and developmental disabilities monitoring network, united states, 2006. *Morbidity and Mortality Weekly Report Surveillance Summaries,* 58(10), 1-20.

Centers for Disease Control and Prevention. (2007a). Prevalence of autism spectrum disorders—autism and developmental disabilities monitoring network, six sites, united states, 2000. *Morbidity and Mortality Weekly Report Surveillance Summaries,* 56(No. SS-1), 1–11.

Centers for Disease Control and Prevention. (2007b). Prevalence of autism spectrum disorders—autism and developmental disabilities monitoring network, 14 sites, united states, 2002. *Morbidity and Mortality Weekly Report Surveillance Summaries,* 56(No. SS-1), 12–28.

* Centers for Disease Control and Prevention. (2007c). Evaluation of a methodology for a collaborative multiple source surveillance network for autism spectrum disorders—autism and developmental disabilities monitoring network, 14 sites, united states, 2002. *Morbidity and Mortality Weekly Report Surveillance Summaries,* 56(No. SS-1), 29–40.

Durkin, M., Maenner, M., Meaney, F., Levy, S., Diguiseppi, C., Nicholas, J., et. al. (2010). Socioeconomic inequality in the prevalence of autism spectrum disorder: evidence from a u.s. cross-sectional study. *PLoS One,* 5(7), e 11551.

Durkin, M., Maenner, M., Newschaffer, C., Lee, L., Cunniff, C., Daniels, J., et al. (2008). Advanced parental age and the risk of autism spectrum disorder. *American Journal of Epidemiology,* 168 (11), 1268–1276.

Giarelli, E., Wiggins, L., Rice, C., Levy, S., Kirby, R., Pinto-Martin, J., et. al. (2010). Sex differences in the evaluation and diagnosis of autism spectrum disorders among children. *Disability and Health Journal,* 3 (2), 107-116.

Kalkbrenner, A., Daniels, J., Chen, J., Poole, C., Emch, M., Morrissey, J. (2010). Perinatal exposure to hazardous air pollutants and autism spectrum disorders at age 8. *Epidemiology,* 21(5), 631-641.

Levy, S., Giarelli, E., Lee, L., Schieve, L., Kirby, R., Cunniff, C., et. al. (2010). Autism spectrum disorders and co-occurring developmental, psychiatric, and medical conditions among children in multiple populations of the united states. *Journal of Developmental and Behavioral Pediatrics,* 31(4), 267-275.

Mandell, D., Wiggins, L., Carpenter, L., Daniels, J., DiGuiseppi, C., Durkin, M., et. al. (2009). Racial/ethnic disparities in the identification of children with autism spectrum disorders. *American Journal of Public Health,* 99(3), 493-498.

* Nonkin Avchen, R., Wiggins, L., Devine, O., Van Naarden-Braun, K., Rice, C., Hobson, N., et. al. (2010).

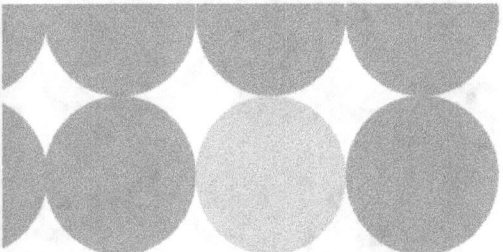

Evaluation of a records-review surveillance system used to determine the prevalence of autism spectrum disorders. *Journal of Autism and Developmental Disorders,* (Epub ahead of print).

Pinborough-Zimmerman, J., Bilder, D., Satterfield, R., Hossain, S., McMahon W. (2010). The impact of surveillance method and record source on autism prevalence: collaboration with utah maternal and child health programs. *Maternal and Child Health Journal,* 14(3), 392-400.

Rice, C., Baio, J., Van Naarden Braun, K., Doernberg, N., Meaney, F., Kirby, R., et. al. (2007). A public health collaboration for the surveillance of autism spectrum disorders. *Paediatric and Perinatal Epidemiology,* 21(2), 179-190.

* Rice, C., Nicholas, J., Baio, J., Pettygrove, S., Lee, L., Van Naarden Braun, K., et. al. (2010). Changes in autism spectrum disorder prevalence in 4 areas of the united states. *Disability and Health Journal,* 3(3), 186-201.

Schieve, L., Baio, J., Rice, C., Durkin, M., Kirby, R., Drews-Botsch, C., et. al. (2010). Risk for cognitive deficit in a population-based sample of u.s. children with autism spectrum disorders: variation by perinatal health factors. *Disability and Health Journal,* 3(3), 202-212.

Van Naarden Braun, K., Schieve, L., Daniels, J., Durkin, M., Giarelli, E., Kirby, R., et al. (2008). Relationships between multiple births and autism spectrum disorders, cerebral palsy, and intellectual disabilities: autism and developmental disabilities monitoring (addm) network—2002 surveillance year. *Autism Research,* 1(5), 265-316.

Trends in Other Conditions

* Atladóttir, H., Parner, E., Schendel, D., Dalsgaard, S., Thomsen, P., Thorsen, P. (2007). Time trends in reported diagnoses of childhood neuropsychiatric disorders: a danish cohort study. *Archives of Pediatrics & Adolescent Medicine,* 161, 193-198.

* Demir, A., Celikel, S., Karakaya, G., Kalyonco, A. (2010). Asthma and allergic diseases in school children from 1992 to 2007 with incidence data. *Journal of Asthma,* 47, 1128-1135.

Finkelhor, D., Turner, H., Ormrod, R., Hamby, S. (2010). Trends in childhood violence and abuse exposure evidence from 2 national surveys. *Archives of Pediatrics & Adolescent Medicine,* 164(3), 238-242.

Ford, E., Ajani, U., Croft, J., Critchley, J., Labarthe, D., Kottke, T. (2007). Explaining the decrease in u.s. deaths from coronary disease, 1980-2000. *The New England Journal of Medicine,* 356, 2388-2398.

Fridkin, S., Hill, H., Volkova, N., Edwards, J., Lawton, R., Gaynes, R., et. al. (2002). Temporal changes in prevalence of antimicrobial resistance in 23 u.s. hospitals. *Emerging Infectious Diseases,* 8(7), 697-701.

* Galea, S. Hall, C., Kaplan, G. (2009). Social epidemiology and complex system dynamic modeling as applied to health behaviour and drug use research. *International Journal on Drug Policy,* 20(3), 209–216.

* Galea, S., Riddle, M., Kaplan, G. (2010). Casual thinking and complex system approaches in epidemiology. *International Journal of Epidemiology,* 39, 97-106.

Hermanussen, M., Danker-Hopfe, H., Weber, G. (2001). Body weight and the shape of the natural distribution of weight, in very large samples of german, austrian and norwegian conscripts. *International Journal of Obesity and Related Metabolic Disorders,* 25(10), 1550-1553.

James, A., Knuiman, M., Divitini, M., Hui, J., Hunter, M., Palmer, L. (2010). Changes in the prevalence of asthma in adults since 1966: the busselton health study. *European Respiratory Journal,* 35, 273-278.

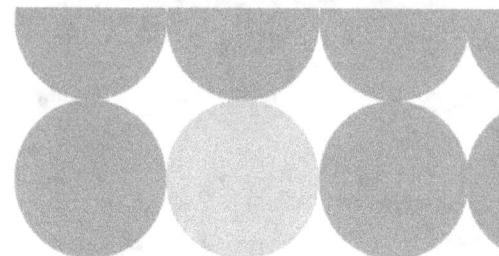

Mandell, D., Thompson, W., Weintraub, E., DeStefano, F., Blank, M. (2005). Trends in diagnosis rates in autism and adhd at hospital discharge in the context of other psychiatric diagnoses. *Psychiatric Services,* 56, 56-62.

* Pallapies, D. (2006). Trends in childhood disease. *Mutation Research,* 608(2), 100-111.

Pastor PN, Reuben CA. (2008). Diagnosed attention deficit hyperactivity disorder and learning disability: United States, 2004–2006. National Center for Health Statistics. Vital Health Stat 10(237).

Robertson, M. (2008). The prevalence and epidemiology of gilles de la tourette syndrome. part 2: tentative explanations for differing prevalence figures in gts, including the possible effects of psychopathology, aetiology, cultural differences, and differing phenotypes. *Journal of Psychosomatic Research*, 65(5), 473–486.

Singh, I. (2006). A framework for understanding trends in adhd diagnoses and stimulant drug treatment: schools and schooling as a case study. *BioSocieties*, 1, 439-452.

Steenland, K., MacNeil, J., Vega, I., Levey, A. (2009). Recent trends in alzheimer's disease mortality in the united states, 1999-2004. *Alzheimer Disease & Associated Disorders*, 23(2), 165-170.

* Van Den Eeden, S., Tanner, C., Bernstein, A., Fross, R., Leimpeter, A., Bloch, D., et. al. (2003). Incidence of parkinson's disease:variation by age, gender, and race/ethnicity. *American Journal of Epidemiology*, 157(11), 1015-1022.

Woodruff, T., Axelrad, D., Kyle, A., Nweke, O., Miller, G., Hurley, B. (2004). Trends in environmentally related childhood illnesses.*Pediatrics*, 113(4), 1133-1140.

Other ASD Prevalence and Epidemiologic Studies

Baird, G., Simonoff, E., Pickles, A., Chandler, S., Loucas, T., Meldrum, D., et al. (2006). Prevalence of disorders of the autism spectrum in a population cohort of children in south thames: the special needs and autism project (SNAP). *Lancet*, 368, 210–215.

* Baron-Cohen, S., Scott, F., Allison, C., Williams, J., Bolton, P., Matthews, F., et al. (2009). Prevalence of autism spectrum conditions: uk school-based population study. *British Journal of Psychiatry*, 194, 500–509.

Bertrand J, Mars A, Boyle C, Bove F, Yeargin-Allsopp M, Decoufle P. (2001). Prevalence of autism in a United States population: The Brick Township, New Jersey, Investigation. *Pediatrics*, 108(5):1155-1161.

Brugha, T., McManus, S., Meltzer, H., Smith, J., Scott, F., Purdon, S., et. al. (2009). Autism spectrum disorders in adults living in households throughout england report from the adult psychiatric morbidity survey 2007. *The Health & Social Care Information Centre, Social Care Statistics*.

* Heussler, H., Polnay, L., Marder, E., Standen, P., Chin, L., Butler, N. (2001). Prevalence of autism in early 1970s may have beenunderestimated. *BMJ*, 323(7313), 633.

Honda, H., Shimizu, Y., Rutter, M. (2005). No effect of mmr withdrawal on the incidence of autism: a total population study. *Journal of Child Psychology and Psychiatry*, 46(6), 572-579.

Kadesjo, B., Gillberg, C., Hagberg, B. (1999). Brief report: autism and asperger syndrome in seven-year-old children: a total population study. *Journal of Autism and Developmental Disorders*, 29(4), 327-331.

* Kogan, M., Blumberg, S., Schieve, L., Boyle, C., Perrin, J. et. al. (2009). Prevalence of parent-reported diagnosis of autism spectrum disorder among children in the U.S., 2007. *Pediatrics*, 124(5), 1395-1403.

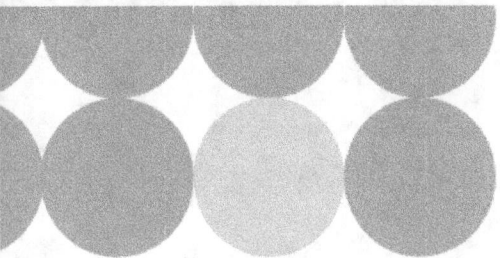

Kuban, K., O'Shea, T., Allred, E., Tager-Flusberg, H., Goldstein, D., Leviton, A. (2009). Positive screening on the modified checklist for autism in toddlers (m-chat) in extremely low gestational age newborns. *Journal of Pediatrics*, 154(4), 535-540.

Nassar, N., Dixon, G., Bourke, J., Bower, C., Glasson, E., de Klerk, N., et. al. (2009). Autism spectrum disorders in young children: effect of changes in diagnostic practices. *International Journal of Epidemiology*, 38(5), 1245-1254.

* Newschaffer, C., Croen, L., Daniels, J., Giarelli, E., Grether, J., Levy, S., et. al. (2007). The epidemiology of the autism spectrum disorders. *Annual Review of Public Health*, 28, 235-258.

Parner, E., Schendel, D., Thorsen. P. (2008). Autism prevalence trends over time in denmark: changes in prevalence and age at diagnosis. *Archives of Pediatrics and Adolescent Medicine*, 162(12), 1150-1156.

* Posserud, M., Lundervold, A., Gillberg, C. (2006). Autistic features in a total population of 7–9-year-old children assessed by the assq (autism spectrum screening questionnaire). *Journal of Child Psychology and Psychiatry, and Allied Disciplines*, 47(2), 167-175.

* Posserud, M., Lundervold, A., Lie, S., Gillberg, C. (2010). The prevalence of autism spectrum disorders: impact of diagnostic instrument and non-response bias. *Social Psychiatry and Psychiatric Epidemiology*, 45(3), 319-327.

Rosenberg, R., Daniels, A., Law, J., Law, P., Kaufmann, W. (2009). Trends in autism spectrum disorder diagnoses: 1994-2007. *Journal of Autism and Developmental Disorders*, 39(8), 1099-1111.

* Saemundsen, E., Juliusson, H., Hjaltested, S., Gunnarsdottir, T. (2010). Prevalence of autism in an urban population of adults with severe intellectual disabilities-a preliminary study. *Journal of Intellectual Disability Research*, 54(8), 727-735.

Thompson L, Kemp J, Wilson P, Pritchett R, Minnis H, Toms-Whittle L, Puckering C, Law J, Gillberg C. (2010). What have birth cohort studies asked about genetic, pre- and perinatal exposures and child and adolescent onset mental health outcomes? A systematic review. *European Child and Adolescent Psychiatry*.,19(1), 1-15.

Treffort, D. (1970). The epidemiology of infantile autism. *Archives of General Psychiatry*, 22, 431-438.

Other Basic Science

Laviola, G., Ognibene, E., Romano, E., Adriani, W., Keller, F. (2009). Gene-environment interaction during early development in the heterozygous reeler mouse: clues for modeling of major neurobehavioral syndromes. *Neuroscience and Biobehavioral Reviews*, 33(4), 560-572.

Van Vliet, J., Oates, N., Whitelaw, E. (2007). Epigenetic mechanisms in the context of complex diseases. *Cellular and Molecular Life Sciences,* 64, 1531 – 1538.

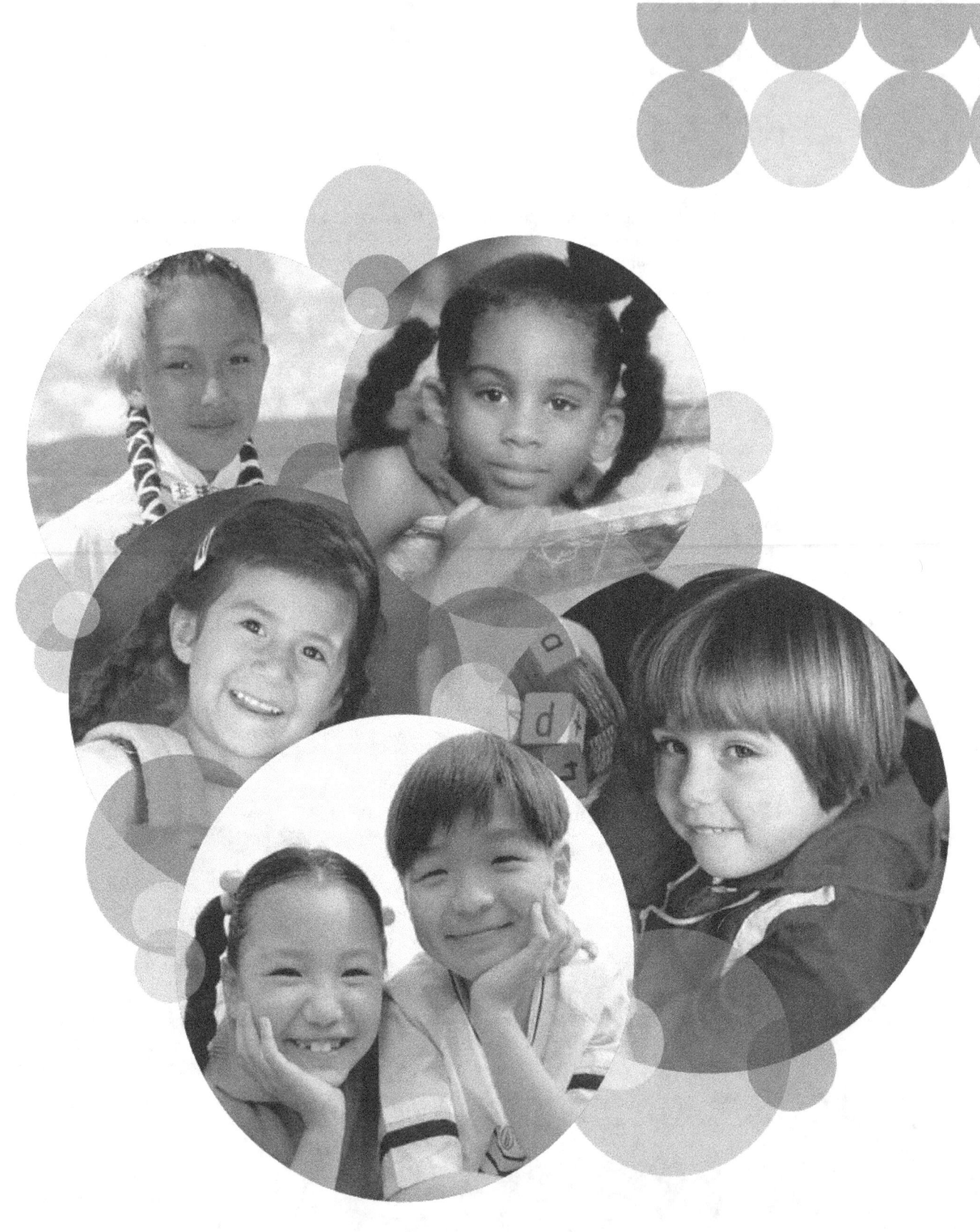

Centers for Disease Control and Prevention
www.cdc.gov/autism
cdcinfo@cdc.gov
1-800-CDC-INFO

Autism Speaks
www.autismspeaks.org
research@autismspeaks.org
1-212-252-8584

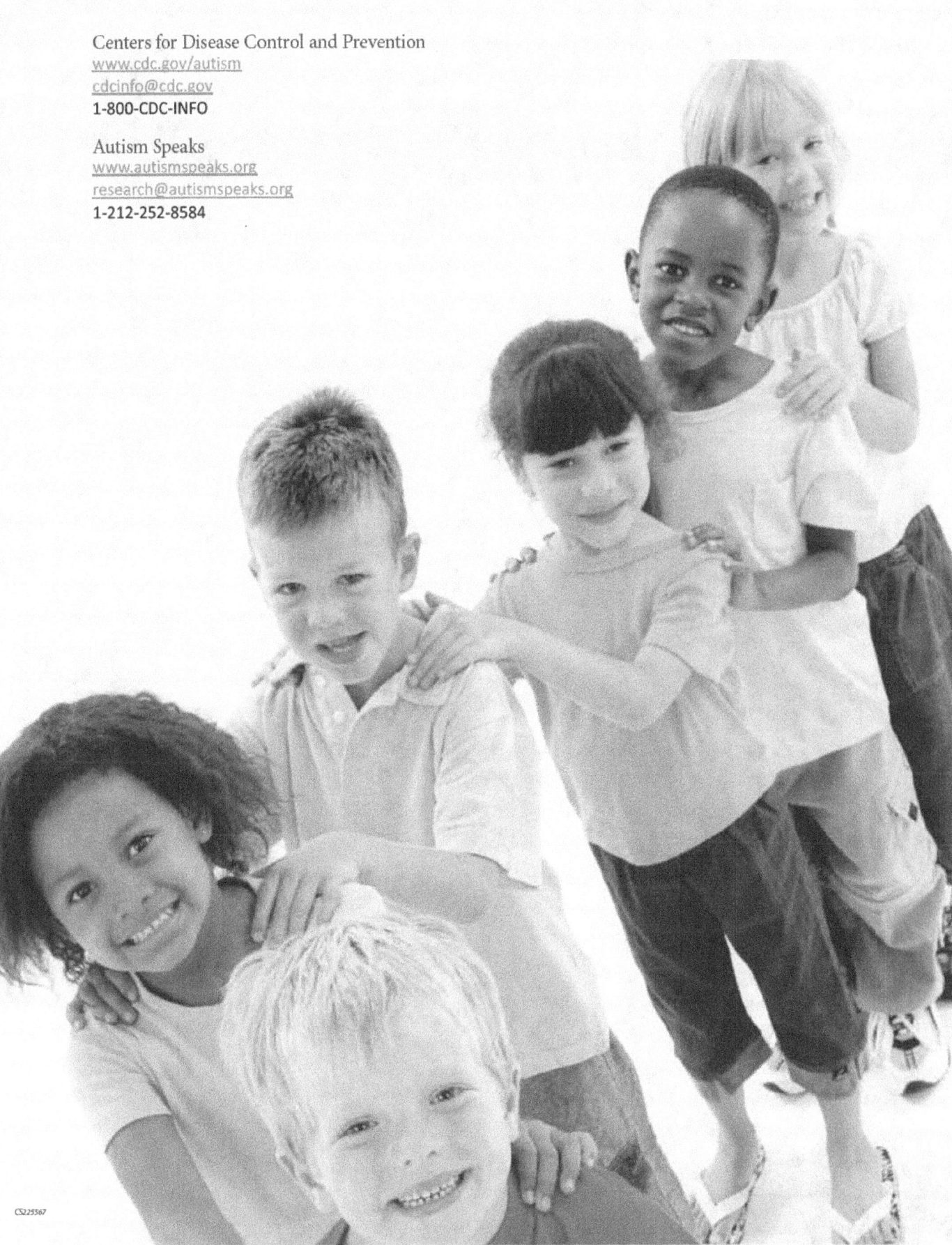

CS225567